Praise for
Models Do Eat

"I love that Jill de Jong is not only taking the fear away from eating, but intelligently guides you in her easy-to-follow book toward delicious and healthy recipes."

—Gabby Reece

"Jill de Jong and her expert coauthors show you not only that models *do* eat—but that nourishing food is what allows them to look and feel as good as they do! This book is packed with beautifying recipes that will inspire you to feed your body well at every meal."

—Jolene Hart, health coach and author of the bestselling Eat Pretty series

"*Models Do Eat* is a great book to use for everyday living. As a model myself, I constantly get asked what do I eat? I'm a firm believer in organic and foods that fuel your body, avoiding diet traps like counting calories or eating fat-free, depriving one's self. This book has the best kind of recipes: easy to follow and powerful for mind, body, and soul."

—Robyn Lawley, *Sports Illustrated* cover model

"Never trust anyone who tells you that not eating is the key to looking good! I applaud Jill and her team for creating this stunning, important book about one of the best parts of life: delicious, nourishing food! *Models Do Eat* is a celebration of healthy eating for real beauty—inside and out."

—Lauren Lobely, author of Accidental Paleo and plant-based chef

"Jill is such an inspiring woman. She's the real deal; she practices what she preaches. I'll always be on team Jill because she genuinely wants everyone to win."

—Nadine Velazquez, actress

"I used to eat lots of processed foods and over-exercised to make up for it. Jill introduced me to eating clean, unprocessed, delicious food, and I discovered that a healthy lifestyle was far from boring. I finally found the balance I needed. Jill has a very light and beautiful way to approach people and I am sure this book and her approach to food will captivate you."

—Martha Graeff, fashion blogger and model

Models Do Eat

Models Do Eat

MORE THAN 100 RECIPES FOR EATING YOUR WAY
TO A BEAUTIFUL, HEALTHY YOU

Jill de Jong

BenBella Books, Inc.
Dallas, TX

Copyright © 2019 by Jill de Jong

"Foreword" © 2019 by Sarah DeAnna
"Less Sugar, More Spice" © 2019 by Taylor Walker Sinning
"Paleo Party" © 2019 by Courtney James
"Simply Delicious" © 2019 by Lauren Williams
"Happy Belly" © 2019 by Colleen Baxter

"Fitness Fuel" © 2019 by Adela Capova
"Unhealthy Foods Made Healthy" © 2019 by Liana Werner-Gray
"Mostly Plants" © 2019 by Summer Rayne Oakes
"Sweets and Treats" © 2019 by Nikki Sharp

Photo credits on page 227.

BenBella
BenBella Books, Inc.
10440 N. Central Expressway, Suite 800
Dallas, TX 75231
www.benbellabooks.com
Send feedback to feedback@benbellabooks.com

Printed in the United States of America
10 9 8 7 6 5 4 3 2 1

Library of Congress Cataloging-in-Publication Data
Names: Jong, Jill de, author.
Title: Models do eat : more than 100 recipes for eating your way to a beautiful, healthy you / Jill de Jong.
Description: Dallas, TX : BenBella Books, Inc., [2019] | Includes bibliographical references and index.
Identifiers: LCCN 2018027320 (print) | LCCN 2018028346 (ebook) | ISBN 9781946885722 (electronic) | ISBN 9781946885517 (trade paper : alk. paper)
Subjects: LCSH: Cooking (Natural foods) | Nutrition. | Natural foods. | Diet. | LCGFT: Cookbooks.
Classification: LCC TX741 (ebook) | LCC TX741 J66 2019 (print) | DDC 641.3/02—dc23
LC record available at https://lccn.loc.gov/2018027320

Editing by Trish Sebben-Malone
Copyediting by Karen Levy
Proofreading by Amy Zarkos and Karen Wise
Indexing by WordCo Indexing Services, Inc.
Text design by Faceout Studios, Paul Nielson

Text composition by Aaron Edmiston
Cover design by Sarah Avinger
Front cover photography by Greg Hinsdale Photography, Inc.; background ©
        Shutterstock / nattha99
Printed by Versa Press

Distributed to the trade by Two Rivers Distribution, an Ingram brand
www.tworiversdistribution.com

Special discounts for bulk sales (minimum of 25 copies) are available. Please contact bulkorders@benbellabooks.com.

Contents

Simply Delicious
BY LAUREN WILLIAMS

Happy Belly
BY COLLEEN BAXTER

Fitness Fuel
BY ADELA CAPOVA

Unhealthy Foods Made Healthy
BY LIANA WERNER-GRAY

Mostly Plants

BY SUMMER RAYNE OAKES

Sweets and Treats

BY NIKKI SHARP

Liquid Recipes

BY JILL DE JONG

Foreword

I'll never forget standing outside my agent's office in Paris and overhearing a conversation between her and another young model, who was sobbing about her weight, measurements, and food choices. My agent specifically told the girl, "You are a model! And models don't eat CHOCOLATE!" I was standing there quietly freaking out. What? Really? Models don't eat chocolate? My life is over if models don't eat chocolate, because chocolate, raw chocolate specifically, is one of my true food pleasures and something I eat nearly every day. This was also the same agent who almost fell off her chair when I told her that I ate a whole bag of cashews for dinner the night before. She said that if I kept that up, I would get fat! Well, I still eat chocolate and cashews, and I'm still a model, and I'm not fat.

The truth is that models eat whatever they want. Models do eat chocolate. And models do eat pizza. And sugar. And all kinds of other foods. We love to eat and most of us also love to cook. Today, we even love to post about it on social media and write books about what to eat and how to eat, because hey, we are models and looking good and feeling good is our job. It's also something we are constantly asked about. People always want to know what we eat, how much we eat, and so on. It often makes me uncomfortable, because a lot of the models and celebrities I advise want to eat exactly what I eat, but healthy eating doesn't work that way. You have to eat what's right for you, not what's right for me or what's right for anyone else in this book.

Besides, just because we are models doesn't mean we're perfect. We have our issues and insecurities. We have days that we are not happy with our bodies, bad hair days, and those really awful days where nothing seems to go right. We don't know everything, but what we do know is how to look our best, how to maintain our ideal body weight, and how to feel good about ourselves inside and out. And just because it's not necessarily your job doesn't mean you can't "model" yourself after a model and in return look and feel like the model version of yourself.

In my book *Supermodel You*, I talk about "mindful eating." It's about getting in tune with your body, eating what you want and when you want, based on what your body is asking for and what it truly needs. Unfortunately, most of us have lost touch with this innate knowing and understanding of our own personal nutrition needs. When we are born, breastfeeding is a natural instinct. I realize that not everyone can or does breastfeed, but I always look at the natural world for what the best thing to do is. In the case of breastfeeding, all signs point to the fact that it is supposed to be our first and most perfect food source. What's also amazing about breastfeeding is that breastfed infants will only feed when they are hungry and stop feeding when they are full.

How, when, and why did we lose touch with the ability to self-regulate our own nutrition and consumption needs? My best guess is that it was when we shut down our internal signals, stopped listening to ourselves, and started giving too much authority to our parents, doctors, nutritionists, friends, the media, marketing,

and so on. Who, more than you, really knows what you need? And I am not just talking about dietary choices here. The question is relevant for all of our life choices.

The book you're holding in your hands is titled *Models Do Eat*, and it's true. We eat a lot. We eat often. And we eat all kinds of different things. I'm excited to be a part of this cookbook collaboration because this is a message I believe in and support. Models have a bad reputation for being stuck up and self-centered, or being drug addicts and having eating disorders. I believe it's important to shine a positive light on models and on our industry because we are so often in the public eye. As you will see in this book, models today are far more likely to be health addicts—addicted to yoga, juicing, and kale chips, rather than drugs or some other unhealthy habit. All the models in this book are successful, inspiring women who love to eat. Not all of us are vegetarians, gluten-free, or follow any specific diet. We eat what's right for us, and in sharing our food choices with you, we hope to inspire you to decide and choose what's best for you as well. *Bon appétit*!

— **Sarah DeAnna**,
model and best-selling author of *Supermodel You*,
a mind/body, health, and inspiration book

A Message from Jill

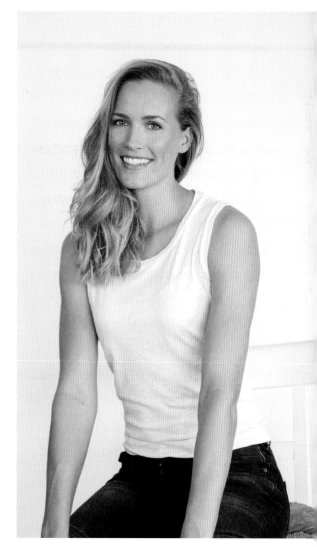

*D*o you love to eat? Do you want to lose weight? Do you want to take better care of yourself? Nine other models and I have put this book together for you! You've probably heard quite a few sad stories about models who smoke cigarettes to suppress their appetite, swallow cotton balls to fake-fill their stomach, or eat low-calorie portions that would barely satisfy a rabbit. And sadly, they're likely true; some models doubtlessly try to meet the demands of the fashion industry in a way that's dangerous and unsustainable. Most models are very young when they get into modeling and simply don't have the right guidance and knowledge.

My coauthors and I can relate to this, as we've all had our own personal challenges staying in shape and dealing with health issues and some forms of disordered eating, which you can read more about at the beginning of each chapter. What we all had in common was a desire to find a better, more enjoyable way to stay fit, healthy, and beautiful. We were looking for answers, and after years of trial and error, we've finally found them!

It's not okay to starve your body—in fact, it's harmful and miserable! Your body needs the best possible nutrition to function properly. Strong nails, shiny hair, and glowing skin are evidence of a good diet. Because good nutrition is all about eating the right things, the search for satisfying yet healthy foods propelled us to do what we do today.

In addition to being models, we are knowledgeable health coaches, trainers, chefs, and authors. In this book, we share our favorite delicious and nutritious recipes that will help you feel and look great! And on top of eating well, we also exercise consistently to stay in shape while striving to take great care of ourselves mentally and spiritually. We want you to know that we are just like you—we deal with insecurities, challenges, and turmoil in our life. If you have bad eating days, bad hair days, bloated and low-energy days, or simply "blah" days, you are not alone!

After many years of international traveling, living in hotels and airplanes, going from one photo shoot to another, and being permanently sleep-deprived, I had recurring health issues that indicated my immune system was weak. I didn't know how to fix it, and I started looking for answers. A visit to a nutritionist was a real eye-opener. He displayed a drop of my blood on a flat-screen TV and explained what was going on inside my body.

I had to eat better: cutting out sugar, eating more veggies and less dairy and bread. There was a lot of room for improvement. But what was I going to eat? If I had to eat better, then healthy food had to taste better; otherwise, it was not going to be sustainable. So, I started looking up simple recipes and taught myself how to cook. I wanted to feel better, have my energy back, and heal my body.

The journey felt empowering and I wanted to share all that I learned with others. I blogged for several years and created many recipes that I envisioned coming together in a book. I worked hard to get the book pitched to publishing houses, and it was disappointing when I only received rejections. But that didn't stop me! I used the rejections as fuel to improve all that I had to offer. I studied at the Institute for Integrative Nutrition and got certified as a heath coach and a personal trainer. In the following years, I helped hundreds of men and women lose weight and improve their health, choices, and mind-set around food and fitness. It's the best job I've ever had.

What will your journey look like? You are an adult. You make your own decisions; you can eat whatever you want, whenever you want. You can eat pie in the morning, a burger for lunch, and pizza for dinner if that's what you desire. But you also know that doing so will not make you feel well, nor will it help you get the fit and healthy body you envision for yourself.

So, let's first focus on our feelings instead of the number on the scale. When you are about to put something in your mouth, ask yourself if it's going to make you feel good. And will that good feeling be temporary or long-lasting? A candy bar might give you some instant satisfaction, but it will inevitably be followed by a sugar crash, making you feel tired and lethargic. A banana, on the other hand, will give you long-lasting energy and keep you mentally focused.

If you have ever been on a diet, you know how restrictive it feels. It sets you up for failure. When you can't have something, you want it even more! If I tell myself I can't eat chocolate for a month, I will think about it all day and dream about it at night. Dieting is no fun; depriving yourself feels like a punishment, right?

And what about the idea that you are "fat"?

The word *fat* holds a lot of power. It has been used for decades to judge ourselves and others in a very unpleasant way. It has caused a lot of tears and unhappiness; being fat has not made anyone popular. Fat people have unfortunately been the target of a lot of jokes, teased, and even beaten up for the size of their body. The emotional scars are real, and recent medical research shows that body weight alone is not an indicator of health—there are plenty of "fat" people who are also fit and healthy for their body type.

There's a lot of confusion and fear around food, resulting in countless people of all ages dealing with some form of disordered eating. Very restrictive and/or uncontrolled eating, such as compulsive overeating, anorexia, bulimia, binge eating, obsessive dieting, and frequent cleansing, are all different types of disordered eating. The modeling industry is often blamed for promoting an unrealistic image of the ideal body, causing women to shame themselves for not having a model-like body. Even though most models naturally have long and lean bodies, they often struggle to maintain it and to meet industry demands.

Luckily, things are slowly changing in the fashion industry. It's wonderful to see a range of sizes on the catwalk and in advertising campaigns. Women of all sizes, colors, and heights are now celebrated. Strong and healthy bodies have never received more attention. And beyond their physical appearance, women of all sizes who are authentic and have something to say to the world are now applauded—a very needed and welcome change!

What would happen if you told yourself that you can eat anything you want, with one condition: that your priority is to make great food choices, because if you do, you'll feel better. Your mind will not feel the need to protest and there will be no resistance—just a quiet resolve to do better for yourself. It's that simple! A new mind-set brings with it a newly adopted lifestyle.

Repeat after me:

"I have the freedom to make my own decisions. I can eat anything I want. My priority is to make good food choices because I want to feel good."

Having freedom of choice is empowering. Depriving or denying yourself isn't.

To make empowering decisions, you need to be well informed. There are so many articles, scientific research papers, and opinions out there on nutrition and exercise. It can be overwhelming, confusing, and sometimes even contradictory. What should you believe?

On the next pages, I'll share my 10 Essentials to help you make better, more informed decisions about your approach to food and nutrition. I wish I had this information presented to me when I was younger, because it has changed my life in the most beneficial way. When you understand the basics of nutrition and how food affects your body, it empowers you to make the best choices for you, every time.

Once we've covered these basics, we'll start cooking. Each chapter highlights a different approach to healthy eating. From protein to Paleo to mostly plant-based, each chapter presents inspiration and recipes for just about any mood, craving, or dietary need. Let this book take you on a little adventure—try new foods and flavor combinations that will dance on your tongue!

It gives me great pleasure to know this book is in your hands. I hope it will inspire you to take charge of your health. When you don't feel good or your health is compromised, you miss out on a lot of fun and beautiful moments in life. Life is precious, and so are you!

Are you ready to enjoy great food and feel better at the same time? Turn the page to start your very own journey to improved health and wellness.

The 10 Essentials

CALORIES

When I was seventeen, I was introduced to calorie counting. I frankly had no clue what a calorie was; the other models in my apartment explained it to me and from that moment on I thought it was my duty to count calories, because that's what professional models did.

For the first time in my life, there was a restriction on the amount of food I could eat. I went to the store to check all the food labels and was not very happy when I noticed that the things I wanted to eat most, like bread, cookies, and chocolate, were high in calories. I wanted to eat, and preferably a lot! I love food. I started exploring diet products; it was a new world in which I could eat a lot of food for fewer calories. Brilliant!

I was snacking all day and skipping a meal here and there—I was figuring it all out. My relationship with food changed. It was all about calories now. When I looked at a menu, I would pick the dish with the least number of calories. I wasn't thinking about what I wanted or what my body needed to be healthy, just picking what I thought was the "better" choice.

I did this for years. Calorie counting took up a lot of headspace, and even though I was eating frequently, I was hungry all day. I was also bloated, gassy, and unhappy. Something had to change.

Most people still think that to lose weight they should eat less and thereby consume fewer calories. Even though it is true that weight loss is caused by a caloric deficit, the "calories in, calories out" model is flawed. If it were really as simple as eating less and moving more, few people would be overweight or bouncing from one diet to the next.

You might think you're outsmarting the system by consuming low-calorie diet products like calorie-free soda and highly processed meal replacements. But what you might not know is that chemicals like artificial sweeteners, flavor enhancers, and preservatives are added to such products to extend their shelf life and make them taste better. And those chemicals can make you overweight and sick.

There are plenty of calorie myths and misconceptions, so let's go back to the drawing board and see if we can understand this important subject better.

A calorie is a measure of energy. The human body requires energy to move, breathe, think, contract the heart, and orchestrate the complex set of chemical reactions that keep us alive. Different foods have different effects on our body and go through different metabolic pathways before they're turned into energy.

Lead researcher Dr. Dariush Mozaffarian, a cardiologist and epidemiologist at the Harvard School of Public Health, says, "What you eat makes quite a difference. Just counting calories won't matter much unless you look at the kinds of calories you're eating."

Your body is a powerful and complex machine. Think of it as a high-performance car. If you were given the choice to put poor-quality or high-quality fuel in the car, wouldn't you choose the latter? Do the same for your body! Pick fuel that provides long-lasting energy, promotes good digestion, and protects your heart. It's important to know that all calories are not created equal.

If you eat 200 calories of raw nuts or a 200-calorie candy bar, do you think your body will process these foods identically? No way! Although they contain the exact same number of calories, your body will react to them very differently. The nuts contain valuable nutrients that nourish your body—the candy bar does not.

I'm not saying that counting calories doesn't work, but it's far more important to worry about the nutrient density of your food than its caloric density. Let me explain the difference: nutrient-dense foods contain high levels of nutrients, such as protein, carbohydrates, fats, vitamins, and minerals, but with fewer calories. These foods provide the most bang for your nutritional buck and include quinoa, berries, kale, sweet potatoes, broccoli, and tomatoes. The great thing about nutrient-dense food is that it keeps you full longer, which in turn will naturally help you eat less.

In contrast, calorie-dense foods contain high levels of calories per serving, often with few healthful benefits. You can say that these foods contain "empty calories," as they provide energy from calories but lack significant nutritional value. It's best to avoid calorie-dense foods and beverages. Many processed foods, such as cakes, cookies, doughnuts, and candies, are considered calorie-dense.

Finally, some foods are a combination of the two. Foods that are nutrient-dense and calorie-dense at the same time include nuts, olive oil, avocado, oily fish, eggs, and whole grains. Even though they're higher in calories, you should still consume these foods in moderation—they're very good for you!

GLUTEN

I was born and raised in Holland, the nation of tall cheese eaters. On average, a Dutch person eats a whopping 18 kilos, or about 39 pounds, of cheese a year! And how do we consume most of that cheese? We love cheese sandwiches. Mind you that in Holland our sandwiches are very simple: a layer of butter and a layer of cheese

on whole-grain bread. When I first came to the States and ordered a cheese sandwich, I wasn't sure what to think of the six layers of cheese on the enormous sandwich in front of me. My goodness, my mouth could hardly fit around the tower of cheese piled with toppings!

In Holland, it's normal to have two bread meals a day. As a teenager, I would consume anywhere between six and ten slices of bread daily. I would eat a few slices before hopping on my bicycle to school, and after that six-mile ride, I would be hungry again, so at lunch I would devour the rest. Eating bread was as ingrained in my daily routine as brushing my teeth.

In my mid-twenties, I went to see a nutritionist; I had several complaints and felt something wasn't right. After a fascinating projection of my blood onto a flat-screen TV, the diagnosis was that I needed a cleanse and probiotics to heal my gut. I was eating healthfully, but the nutrients weren't properly absorbed because bad bacteria were populating my gut. Part of the cleanse required not eating gluten for six weeks. My body was in utter shock; never in my life had I gone that long without eating bread, pasta, and other wheat products! It was hard to find good substitutes; I felt hungry and empty all day and night.

Thank God it wasn't a life sentence, though—I wasn't gluten intolerant. My body just needed a break, and I learned that yes, fewer wheat products would be better. I now have plenty of great gluten-free foods in my regular diet and still enjoy bread and other products with gluten, just less frequently than I used to.

You see and hear a lot about gluten and gluten-free products, but what is gluten, exactly? Gluten is the name of one of the proteins in barley, rye, and all forms of wheat. It's the protein found in wheat that gives elasticity to dough, helping it rise and keep its shape while baking.

The market for gluten-free products is exploding. Many people may perceive that a gluten-free diet is healthy. But don't be fooled—a food labeled as "gluten-free" isn't necessarily healthy at all! There might not be gluten in your cupcake, but it's probably still high in calories, fat, and sugar.

Experts estimate that about 6 percent of Americans suffer from some level of gluten intolerance or wheat allergies, while only 1 percent have celiac disease, a hereditary autoimmune condition that causes an abnormal immune response to gluten that damages the lining of the small intestine. This damage to the digestive tract can prevent important nutrients from being absorbed and can trigger many other troublesome health issues.

Celiac disease symptoms include bloating, abdominal pain, lethargy, brain fog, and anxiety. If you experience these symptoms after eating gluten, you may want to get tested for celiac. Or you can go gluten-free for a week or two to see if you feel any different, and then slowly add gluten back into your diet. Going gluten-free temporarily may also inspire you to eat a wider variety of foods, and you may even lose a few pounds!

A permanent gluten-free diet is only for those who are sensitive to, or intolerant of, gluten. And if you consider yourself gluten-sensitive (not intolerant), look at the quality of the barley, rye, and wheat products you consume. Are you eating processed white bread and pasta, or are you eating the whole-grain and sprouted versions? It could be the white flour and chemicals in your food making you feel bloated and lethargic.

A gluten-free diet can lack vitamins, minerals, and fiber. Gluten itself doesn't offer special nutritional benefits, but the many whole grains that contain gluten do. They're rich in an array of vitamins and minerals, such as B vitamins and iron, as well as fiber. But if you must cut gluten out of your diet, don't panic! A few whole grains such as amaranth, millet, and quinoa are naturally gluten-free and provide a wealth of nutrients.

THE GLUTEN-FREE SHOPPING LIST

Yum!

Run!

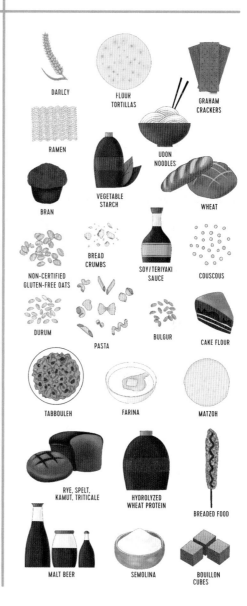

Yum! column:

- BEANS, PEAS & LEGUMES
- SPICES
- EGGS
- CHEESE
- POTATO
- BUTTER
- NUTS
- SORGHUM
- SEEDS
- FLAXSEED
- FRUITS
- VEGETABLES
- FISH & MEATS
- YOGURT
- CORN
- QUINOA
- YEAST
- TAPIOCA
- BUCKWHEAT
- RICE
- MILLET
- SOY
- OILS
- VANILLA EXTRACT
- MILK
- VEG. BROTH
- TAMARI

Run! column:

- BARLEY
- FLOUR TORTILLAS
- GRAHAM CRACKERS
- RAMEN
- UDON NOODLES
- VEGETABLE STARCH
- WHEAT
- BRAN
- NON-CERTIFIED GLUTEN-FREE OATS
- BREAD CRUMBS
- SOY / TERIYAKI SAUCE
- COUSCOUS
- DURUM
- PASTA
- BULGUR
- CAKE FLOUR
- TABBOULEH
- FARINA
- MATZOH
- RYE, SPELT, KAMUT, TRITICALE
- HYDROLYZED WHEAT PROTEIN
- BREADED FOOD
- MALT BEER
- SEMOLINA
- BOUILLON CUBES

Keeping a food diary is a good way to monitor how your body responds to the food you eat. Write down what you eat and drink all day and how you feel after consuming it. Do you feel tired or energized after lunch? Do you feel short-tempered or relaxed? You might discover some food-mood connections, which can also help you figure out if eating gluten is right for you.

CARBS

Most of my clients feel guilty after consuming carbs. I often hear, "I fell off the wagon," "I've been bad," or "I'm mad at myself for giving in." They think that they should be on a no- to low-carb diet to drop pounds. And not only do they feel bad about eating carbs, but they feel even worse reporting it to me. I listen to their self-shaming and then, after a brief silence, I ask kindly, "I hope you enjoyed it? And how did you feel afterward?" Somewhat confused, expecting me to disapprove of their choice, they recall that moment of eating the carbs and then the hours afterward.

Most of the time I hear that they didn't feel great after the meal. "Tired and bloated" are probably the most common words they use to describe the aftermath of a carb feast. I like them to think about those feelings, because when something tastes

good for a few minutes but makes you feel unwell for hours afterward, it's often not worth eating again. I love carbs and eat my fair share daily; the amount depends on how active I am. Carbs make me feel nourished, satiated, and energized. But it's all about picking the right carbs—the ones that work for you, not against you.

Everyone needs carbohydrates. When you eat carbohydrates, such as breads, pasta, rice, fruits, and vegetables, they are converted into blood glucose to provide immediate energy and then converted into glycogen for later use. If you eat more calories than you expend, carbohydrates are also converted into stored fat.

When you cut them out altogether, you might lose some weight, but there's a good chance you will also feel tired and cranky. Not ideal! Eating the right kind of carbs is the key to feeling ener-gized and happy, and yes, even losing weight. But what is the right kind?

Complex versus Simple Carbohydrates

Complex (or whole) carbohydrates are predom-inantly plant-based foods that grow in nature. Complex carbohydrate foods contain fiber, vitamins, and minerals, and they take longer to digest, which means they have less of an immediate impact on blood sugar while giving you long-lasting energy.

EXAMPLES: brown rice, quinoa, whole-grain pasta, sweet potatoes, beans, veggies, fresh fruit

Simple (processed) carbohydrates are derived from grains and other plants, but they have been processed and stripped of their fiber. Many refined carbs also have added sugar. They are quickly digested due to their lack of intact fiber, leading to a faster rise in blood sugar, which can have negative health effects. This fast-released energy is stored as glycogen in your cells. And when that stored energy isn't used, it gets converted into fat.

EXAMPLES: candy, doughnuts, pastries, white rice, white pasta, white bread

Obviously, complex carbs are the way to go! But how much should you eat? Everyone is different, and you can identify your optimal carb intake based on how active you are and your fitness goals, existing body composition, and genetics. According to the National Academy of Medicine, adult women should consume 45 to 65 percent of their daily calories from carbohydrates. According to the American Academy of Orthopaedic Surgeons, women athletes may require as many as 60 to 70 percent of their calories from carbs.

Carbohydrates are in most foods, from table sugar, candy, and doughnuts to whole-grain pasta and blueberries. You'll want to pick the healthiest representatives of this food group with smart choices like whole grains, beans, veggies, sweet potatoes, and fresh fruit. Look for labels like "sprouted" or "whole grain" when choosing nutrient-dense bread, pasta, and rice, and avoid the processed, nutrient-stripped, white flour versions.

The bottom line? It's fine to enjoy carbs, as long as you do it the right way. It always makes me happy when clients make better decisions and feel the impact it has on their body and mind. The main reason my clients sign up for health coaching is weight loss. It's wonderful to be part of their journey; the weight comes off naturally, and by changing what they eat and how they move, they enjoy so many other benefits. As for me, I'm not constantly bloated anymore. I sleep much better and feel energized all day. And feeling great is priceless. Happiness is eating carbs without gaining unwanted weight!

PROTEIN

When I first started modeling, I moved to Milan, where I lived with other models in so-called model apartments. This might sound exclusive and luxurious, but trust me—there was nothing glamorous about it. Sharing bedrooms, bathrooms, and a fridge is not exactly ideal for a bunch of foreign girls with busy schedules. These arrangements are common for models everywhere; in New York, I shared a tiny bedroom with three other girls and we slept in bunk beds. There was not even enough space to put our clothes in the closet, so we lived out of our suitcases.

In Milan, I shared an apartment with a Dutch model whom I looked up to. She was more experienced and kindly shared her "do's and don'ts" of the industry with me. She was dating a handsome, muscular, Italian playboy, and he had told her that she needed lots of protein to get in great shape. The best and cheapest way? She ate lots of canned tuna on dry crackers. I had never had tuna before, but I gave it a try and thought it was pretty tasty. It was convenient, too; I didn't know

how to cook back then, so anything out of a can or ready to go was a bonus. I cringe when I think back about eating the same boring thing every day—it was functional, but not enjoyable, and I really didn't know any better! Luckily, I do know better now; there are so many more delicious ways to eat quality protein.

Twenty percent of the human body is made up of protein. Protein plays an important role in most biological processes, and amino acids are the building blocks of it. Their most important task is to store and transport nutrients to the right places. Amino acids also influence the function of organs, glands, tendons, and arteries. Of the twenty amino acids that make up your body's protein, nine are essential to your diet because your cells can't manufacture them. Those nine amino acids should be in your food every day because, unlike fat and starch, the human body doesn't store amino acids for later use.

It's no secret that protein is a woman's best friend. It helps build strong, toned muscles; keeps your hair, skin, and nails beautiful; and helps you feel less hungry because protein-rich food keeps you full longer. No wonder there's so much hype about high-protein diets everywhere! We can't seem to get enough of it. But more is not always better.

Research has found that too much protein can lead to weight gain, overstressed kidneys, osteoporosis, elevated blood sugar, and dehydration. And the type and quality of protein that you consume are important, too.

Most American adults eat more protein than they need, mostly from animal sources. And unfortunately, it's usually in the form of low-quality processed red meat, which has been associated with cancer and cardiovascular disease. Limiting your red meat intake is certainly healthier! Instead, choose high-quality chicken, fish, eggs, and dairy products. You can recognize high-quality products by labels such as "grass-fed," "wild-caught," "organic," "no antibiotics," and "nitrate-free."

You can also choose the often forgotten but oh-so-powerful plant proteins. Your body will benefit greatly from eating more of these. Unlike animal proteins, most plant proteins don't contain all nine vital amino acids. (Some exceptions are quinoa, buckwheat, and soy.) But that's not a deal breaker, as consuming a wide variety of plant proteins, such as wheat, brown rice, corn, peanut butter, beans and legumes, and soy products, will provide your body with a full spectrum of essential amino acids, delivering nutritious protein without the drawbacks of animal products. It's

not necessary to combine plant proteins in every bite or every meal, either. You only need a sufficient amount of each amino acid every day, and if you eat a good variety of foods, it's very likely you'll get enough. To sum it up: eat less animal protein and more plant protein, and always get the best-quality food you can find!

How much protein should you eat daily? That depends on your weight and activity level. See the guidelines for women below:

NOT VERY ACTIVE:
your weight in lb. × 0.36

ACTIVE:
your weight in lb. × 0.5

VERY ACTIVE / ATHLETES:
your weight in lb. × 0.7

For example, let's say you exercise two or three times a week and weigh 140 pounds. You'll need: 140 lb. × 0.5 = 70 grams of protein daily.

Protein doesn't have to be a confusing topic. Now that you know how much you need, take a look at the protein chart, pick your favorite protein sources, and add up the numbers of grams. Consider your daily goal when planning meals.

PLANT-BASED PROTEIN

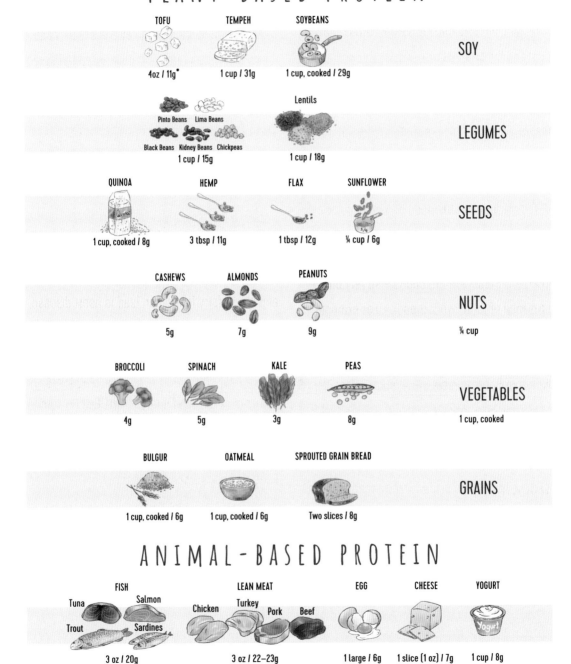

SOY
TOFU — 4oz / 11g*

TEMPEH — 1 cup / 31g

SOYBEANS — 1 cup, cooked / 29g

LEGUMES
Pinto Beans Lima Beans

Black Beans Kidney Beans Chickpeas

1 cup / 15g

Lentils — 1 cup / 18g

SEEDS
QUINOA — 1 cup, cooked / 8g

HEMP — 3 tbsp / 11g

FLAX — 1 tbsp / 12g

SUNFLOWER — ¼ cup / 6g

NUTS
CASHEWS — 5g

ALMONDS — 7g

PEANUTS — 9g

¼ cup

VEGETABLES
BROCCOLI — 4g

SPINACH — 5g

KALE — 3g

PEAS — 8g

1 cup, cooked

GRAINS
BULGUR — 1 cup, cooked / 6g

OATMEAL — 1 cup, cooked / 6g

SPROUTED GRAIN BREAD — Two slices / 8g

ANIMAL-BASED PROTEIN

FISH
Tuna Salmon

Trout Sardines

3 oz / 20g

LEAN MEAT
Chicken Turkey Pork Beef

3 oz / 22–23g

EGG
1 large / 6g

CHEESE
1 slice (1 oz) / 7g

YOGURT
1 cup / 8g

* Number of grams refers to amount of protein per stated serving.

FAT

For years, our relationship status with fat has been complicated, but dietary fat is finally getting the respect it deserves. For decades, we were told that eating fat would make us fat. We feared eating fat and were obsessed with low-fat diets and fat-free and low-fat products—but those dark days are finally over! We now know that fat is an important part of a healthy diet.

Fat is as essential to your diet as protein and carbohydrates are in fueling your body with energy. Certain body functions also rely on the presence of fat to work properly. For example, some vitamins require fat in order to dissolve into your bloodstream and provide your body with nutrition. An adequate amount of healthy fat in your diet also keeps your skin supple and soft. But it's easy to get confused about good fats versus bad fats, so here's a quick overview.

AVOID Trans Fat

The worst type of fat is known as trans fat. Eating artificial trans fat has been shown to raise your "bad" cholesterol levels while lowering your "good" cholesterol levels, leading to an increased risk of heart disease. Trans fats are found in processed foods, and while many brands are choosing not to use it anymore, it's still your responsibility to know what you're putting in your mouth. If you do choose to eat processed foods, don't skip reading the ingredient list on the label. Trans fat is typically listed as "partially hydrogenated oil." Suspect food items include doughnuts, cookies, pancake mix, muffins, pies, and cakes. Some restaurants and fast-food outlets still use cheap trans fats to deep-fry foods, too.

LIMIT Saturated Fat

For decades, we've been warned that eating saturated fat, the type found in eggs, meat, cheese, and many dairy foods, can lead to heart disease, but new research suggests otherwise. Not everyone agrees that saturated fats are totally harmless, but it's safe to say that consuming small amounts of this food group is fine. Just be sure to get the best quality you can afford by choosing organic, grass-fed meats and pasture-raised dairy and eggs whenever possible.

Coconut oil is another saturated fat, but one that is considered healthy when consumed in moderation. According to Livestrong.com, the saturated fat in coconut oil is not like that found in animal products. Coconut oil is a medium-chain fatty acid, while animal fats are long-chain fatty acids. Medium-chain fatty acids are used directly by the body to create energy. They may not negatively affect cholesterol and may also help reduce your risk of heart disease.

ENJOY Unsaturated Fats and Omega-3 Fatty Acids

There's plenty of room in your diet for "good fats"! Unlike trans fats, unsaturated fats and omega-3 fatty acids can help lower cholesterol and protect against heart disease. The amount of good fat you should consume daily is still a controversial topic; the current guideline is between 20 and 30 percent of your total daily calorie intake. Use common sense: enjoy a handful of nuts, snack on half an avocado, put a tablespoon or two of olive oil on salads, and eat fatty fish twice a week.

Eating fat won't make you fat! It's vital for satiation, high energy levels, glowing skin, and improved brain function. Just make sure you're eating the right kinds of fat and always choose the highest quality.

SUGAR

A new client came to me with a list of worrisome symptoms. This young mother was extremely tired and scattered, with headaches and near-constant indigestion. She had been

NUTS

walnuts, macadamia, Brazil, peanuts, cashews, almonds, pistachios

SEEDS

chia, flax, hemp, sunflower, sesame, pumpkin

VEGETABLES

avocados and omega-3-rich cruciferous vegetables, such as broccoli, kale, cauliflower, Brussels sprouts

FATTY FISH

mackerel, lake trout, herring, sardines, albacore tuna, salmon

OILS

extra-virgin olive, palm, fish, krill, flaxseed; always buy high-quality, cold-pressed, and expeller-pressed oils

diagnosed with fibromyalgia, a condition that caused nagging pain in her body. We started with a fridge and pantry makeover, eliminating the most unnatural and processed foods from her diet and making a list of her favorite unhealthy products so that we could swap them out for more nutritious choices. Her husband was excited for the family to get healthier and joined us on our health food store field trip. We walked through all the aisles, reading labels and finding the best-quality products, and purchased a few new foods to try as well.

My client was not confident in the kitchen and therefore didn't enjoy cooking. We began our work by cooking simple, delicious meals together that she proudly served to her family. The kids loved it—they were sipping on smoothies and eating new snacks with gusto. Implementing new habits isn't always easy, but it's so worth it. After a few months of weekly visits, cooking sessions, and coaching with me, eating healthy became this family's new normal. The big reward? My client's symptoms all disappeared, including the pain!

One day I arrived at her house with groceries, as we were planning to cook up a storm. She opened the door looking very ill. She said, "Jill, I'm feeling awful today. I went to one of my children's birthday parties yesterday and ate candy, cake, and hot dogs. The inflammation in my body that was causing the pain is back! I can hardly believe I used to feel like this every day, and even though I'm sick right now, I'm happy to know what caused it and what I can do to feel better." Such teachable moments make me very happy, because as a health coach my goal is to help my clients feel empowered in making the best decisions for themselves.

Implementing new habits is not a linear learning process. It often comes with ups and downs. You might go from one extreme to another before you eventually find a balanced and pleasurable new way of doing things. Even though we know sugar isn't doing us much good, we may find it hard to cut back. Scientists have found that sugar is addictive and stimulates the same pleasure centers in the brain as cocaine or heroin. No wonder we are drawn to eating it! And even though the short sugar high is inevitably followed by a crash, we can't help but crave more.

I challenge you to go sugar-free for a week. Why? To see how you feel! I bet you are going to feel better, and feeling better is the key to sticking with new habits. Let me warn you that during the first few days you might experience some withdrawal symptoms, including anger, anxiety, cravings, fatigue, headaches, and mood swings. But hang in there—it's worth it! Very likely you will soon enjoy benefits such as weight loss, increased energy and mental clarity, better digestion, and a healthy, glowing complexion.

When I say "sugar-free," I mean no added sugar. You already know that you can find sugar in sodas, cookies, desserts, and so on. But how about the added sugar in not-so-obvious foods like flavored yogurts, bottled salad dressings, bread, peanut butter, and cereals? Added sugar is everywhere, used in approximately 75 percent of packaged foods purchased in the United States! It's important to start reading food labels to look for sugar in disguise. It can go by names like corn syrup, evaporated cane juice, glucose, fructose, or malt syrup.

Sugar is often the cause of chronic inflammation, a condition that is associated with heart disease, diabetes, arthritis, and cancer. Consuming excessive amounts of sugar can set off an avalanche of negative health events, both mental and physical. Knowing all this, are you ready to take on the challenge of eliminating sugar from your diet?

During your sugar-free week, a little preparation and determination will help you succeed. Plan to eat breakfast every day, to give your body something nutritious to convert into energy. Eat frequently—three meals a day plus a few healthy snacks will help balance your blood sugar. Finally, eat plenty of veggies as well as some fruit. This will keep you satiated and prevent sugar cravings.

What about artificial sweeteners? They are also banned during Sugar-Free Week, as they are manmade and not naturally occurring in food. If you really need something sweet in your tea or coffee, try a little raw honey. Are you up for the challenge? It's only seven days out of your life, but it could be life-changing!

7-DAY SUGAR-FREE CHALLENGE PREP

- Stock your kitchen with plenty of fresh fruit, vegetables, and whole foods.
- Drink a teaspoon of raw, unfiltered apple cider vinegar diluted in a glass of water twice a day to help curb sweet cravings and level out your blood sugar.
- Keep some naturally sweet dried, unsulfured fruit like dates, raisins, and mango handy for sugar withdrawal emergencies (make sure your dried fruit has no added sugars).

PH: WHAT'S YOUR NUMBER?

An acidic body is an unhealthy body. It's a typical condition in the United States because the Standard American Diet (SAD) contains a large amount of highly acid-forming foods, like meat, dairy, corn, processed wheat, and refined sugars.

When the body is acidic, it creates an unwholesome environment where illness-causing bacteria, fungus, and yeast thrive. Some signs of an acidic body are chronic yeast infections, getting sick frequently, gaining weight, feeling tired, headaches, and premature aging.

I ask my clients to keep a food diary, which is a great way to identify their most consumed acid-forming foods and beverages. The three most common acid-promoting foods are coffee, sugar, and meat. They often eat these foods daily and find them to be quite addictive. I've heard it plenty of times: "I'm happy to change my diet, but don't touch my coffee!"

Change is lasting when it comes from the heart; real growth is possible when you decide you want to do this for yourself and not for anybody else. To encourage such change, I ask my clients if they are interested in doing a little experiment in the best free laboratory in the world, their body. "What if we do a little experiment this week and see how you cope with two cups of joe a day instead of four? You can still drink coffee, just a little less. Let's see what happens!" Cutting down doesn't feel as threatening as quitting altogether, so they're usually willing to take on the challenge.

My clients often discover that eating so much of these damaging foods is merely a habit—it's not something they need as much as they initially thought. In fact, they feel so much better cutting down that it makes them curious what it would feel like to not have any at all. A celebrity client of mine went cold turkey on a film shoot after discovering how much better he felt after drinking less coffee. It was a very demanding shoot, requiring long days and nights on set. He wanted to perform at his best, feeling energized and laser focused. We made sure his diet included plenty of alkalizing fruits and vegetables, and it worked! He was so excited to tell me that it felt as if a fog had lifted. His eye bags disappeared, and he woke up feeling alert and rested instead of groggy.

Your blood should typically have a balanced pH level of about 7.3. This number indicates an alkaline environment with which your body performs optimally. Anything lower than that means your body is acidic and imbalanced. This can cause you to feel tired and sluggish, get sick frequently, and even gain weight despite exercising and watching your food intake. Long term, high acidity can wreak havoc on your health. New research even shows that cancer thrives in an acidic environment and can't survive in an alkaline environment!

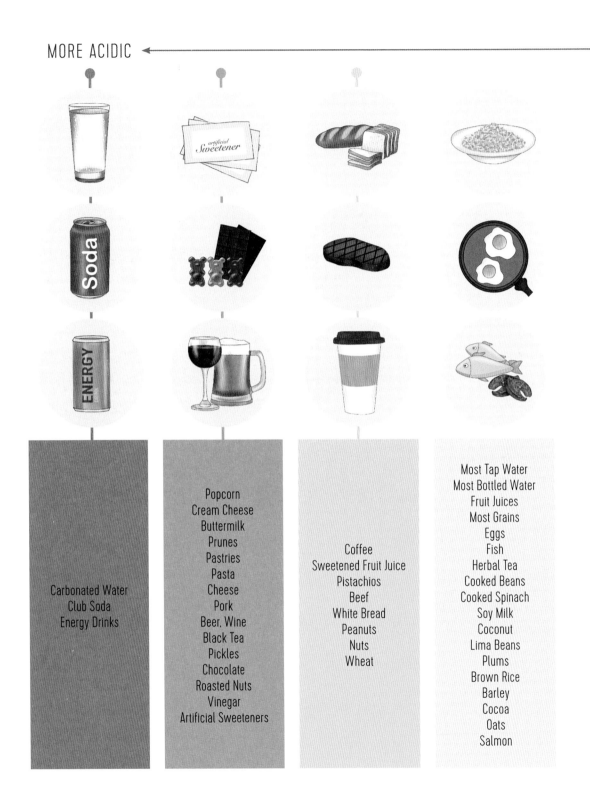

Carbonated Water
Club Soda
Energy Drinks

Popcorn
Cream Cheese
Buttermilk
Prunes
Pastries
Pasta
Cheese
Pork
Beer, Wine
Black Tea
Pickles
Chocolate
Roasted Nuts
Vinegar
Artificial Sweeteners

Coffee
Sweetened Fruit Juice
Pistachios
Beef
White Bread
Peanuts
Nuts
Wheat

Most Tap Water
Most Bottled Water
Fruit Juices
Most Grains
Eggs
Fish
Herbal Tea
Cooked Beans
Cooked Spinach
Soy Milk
Coconut
Lima Beans
Plums
Brown Rice
Barley
Cocoa
Oats
Salmon

ACID / ALKALINE FOOD CHART

Apples	Avocados	Spinach
Almonds	Green Tea	Broccoli
Tomatoes	Lettuce	Artichokes
Grapefruits	Celery	Brussels Sprouts
Corn	Peas	Cabbage
Mushrooms	Sweet Potatoes	Cauliflower
Turnips	Eggplant	Carrots
Olives	Green Beans	Cucumbers
Soybeans	Beets	Lemons
Peaches	Blueberries	Limes
Bell Peppers	Pears	Seaweed
Pineapples	Grapes	Asparagus
Cherries	Kiwis	Kale
Wild Rice	Melons	Radish
Apricots	Tangerines	Collard Greens
Strawberries	Figs	Onions
Bananas	Dates	
	Mangoes	
	Papayas	

Cancer is second on the list of leading causes of death in America and predicted to become number one very soon. It's not surprising that the Standard American Diet (SAD), which consists mainly of foods that are acid-forming (meat, dairy, fish, eggs, sugar, soda, coffee, alcohol, processed food), is a major contributor to rising cancer rates. That's not to say you should stop eating these items, but you should strive to eat them a lot less often. As with most things in life, it's all about finding a healthy balance.

Do you want to know your own pH number? Is your body acidic or alkaline? Just as you would test the pH in a pool, now you can test your body with pH test strips, available on Amazon or www.phreshproducts.com. Improve your alkalinity by following a diet that includes whole foods like lemons and fresh vegetables. Take a look at the acid/alkaline food comparison chart on pages 32–33 and make it a rule of thumb to fill your plate with at least 50 percent (or, optimally, 75 percent) alkaline food.

Reducing acid-forming foods in your diet while increasing alkalizing ones gives your body a chance to restore balance at the cellular level, which allows it to start breaking down fat stores and ultimately rebalance your natural healthy weight.

FIVE WAYS TO SAFELY ALKALIZE YOUR BODY

1. Eat more veggies, especially leafy greens.

2. Eat whole grains like quinoa, spelt, buckwheat groats, and millet.

3. Drink copious amounts of purified water with fresh lemon juice.

4. Drink apple cider vinegar daily. Dilute 1 teaspoon in a glass of water.

5. Get a daily dose of spirulina or raw greens powder by adding it to smoothies or sauces.

WHY ORGANIC?

I was raised in a small village in Holland by parents who did things differently than most families. They were concerned about the environment and very health conscious. My father juiced carrots, listened to meditation music, read self-help books, and did yoga-like stretching way before it became a trend. The apple doesn't fall far from the tree! As a little girl I wasn't always happy with my parents' approach; we had to slice our own bread, which often resulted in thick and ugly slices. Machine-sliced bread was so much cooler! Also, no soft margarine for us; we used hard butter that made holes in the bread when we tried to spread it evenly. One day my parents decided to sell our car. They wanted to save the planet and not pollute it any longer. Instead, we used our bicycles and public transportation to go everywhere.

A mile away from our house we had a community vegetable garden where we grew things like kale, potatoes, green beans, and berries. I had my own little piece that I maintained with much care. My favorite time of the year was when the strawberries were ripe and the carrots big enough to be pulled out of the ground. It was normal in our house to enjoy fresh, seasonal produce. But at some point, the community garden closed down; houses were built, and we didn't have access to a vegetable garden any longer. We began purchasing our produce at the farmers' market or supermarket. We never questioned the quality of the produce—the farmers were people like us and we trusted them.

In retrospect, for a large chunk of my childhood, we were consuming chemically sprayed (nonorganic) produce. The farmers were introduced to a modern way to grow crops and do their business and didn't think the fertilizers or pesticides were harmful to the consumer—after all, they ate it themselves! Little did we know about the long-term health effects of these toxic chemicals. Even though my father is health conscious, it's been hard for him to change; he's been going to that farmers' market for so many years. I believe that this change is particularly hard because he can't physically see the harmful chemicals on his food.

What if you could see the more than forty different toxic pesticides on that conventionally grown apple you're about to eat? You wouldn't want to eat it, right? But because the pesticides aren't visible to the naked eye and because conventional produce looks like, or sometimes even better than, its organic competition, why should you pay extra?

A study published by the *American Journal of Clinical Nutrition* investigated the nutrient content of organic versus conventional foods. The results showed no evidence that organic foods are more nutritious than conventionally grown foods. Does this mean we should not bother buying organic? NO! It might not have a higher nutrient content, but conventional produce may contain plenty of harmful chemicals that could outweigh its nutritional value.

I personally think organic food is much more flavorful, and it's only natural to eat food that is chemically untreated. However, organic food is usually significantly more expensive than conventional food. Many of us can't afford to buy all organic all the time, but we can still reduce the risk of health problems.

Each year, the Environmental Working Group (ewg.org) publishes the Dirty Dozen and the Clean Fifteen lists (page 37) to help us make more informed choices about when to buy organic instead of conventional produce. The column on the left side, the Dirty Dozen, are the fruits and veggies that are most contaminated by pesticide use and therefore best to buy organic. If you can't afford to buy everything organic, look at the Clean Fifteen—these are the least contaminated, so conventionally grown is generally a safe choice. The list is updated every year, so check annually and choose carefully according to your budget.

Removing the skins of fruits and vegetables helps get rid of much of their external chemical residue, but don't forget that they were likely grown in polluted soil to begin with. If you are unsure whether your produce is organic or not, check the PLU code on the sticker to determine its origin—conventionally grown produce has a four-digit code that starts with 3 or 4, while organic produce has a five-digit code that always starts with 9. Do you want more and cheaper organic food available for everyone? Use your purchasing power! Every dollar you spend on organic food helps create a larger demand for chemical-free products. Together, we can change the industry, so shop wisely.

EXERCISE

I was an active child. I had a lot of energy and was good at most sports. I loved games, was very competitive, and was always one of the first to be chosen for a team at school. As a child, exercise was all about having fun. That changed when I started modeling.

My agency wanted me to lose a few inches around my waist, so I went to the gym and asked a trainer what exercises he would recommend. I completed all the rounds of exercises in no time. You should have seen his face when I asked him for more—I was so eager! Going to the gym became part of my job; it was even written into my modeling contract that it was my responsibility to maintain the shape I was in when I signed. If I didn't, I'd run the risk of not working and losing my contract. It may sound

DIRTY DOZEN | CLEAN FIFTEEN

Strawberries

Spinach

Avocados

Sweet Corn

Pineapples

Nectarines

Apples

Cabbage

Onions

Sweet Peas

Grapes

Peaches

Papayas

Asparagus

Mangoes

Cherries

Pears

Eggplant

Honeydew

Kiwis

Tomatoes

Celery

Cantaloupes

Cauliflower

Broccoli

Potatoes

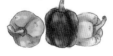

Bell Peppers

kind of crazy, but it's true; there are very few occupations in this world that can legally fire you for being out of shape!

I went to the gym religiously and thought it was a great place to hang out, especially because there were a lot of handsome boys there. An agent noticed that I started to get very toned and told me to exercise less. He wasn't the first one to tell me that; several clients had complained about my visibly toned arms. They wanted no definition, just skinny arms. I reluctantly stopped working out my arms and started exercising less. Other people's opinions can really impact how you feel about your body. You start labeling your body as good or bad, or beautiful or ugly, instead of healthy or unhealthy.

A big shift in my thinking happened when I decided to pursue my passion for health and fitness as a coach and trainer. I stopped caring what agents and clients thought of my body. I was curious to see how my body would develop during training for a triathlon, doing high-intensity interval training (HIIT) and lots of yoga. To my surprise, I didn't bulk up, nor did I shrink. I was simply getting stronger and more defined. The funny thing is that nowadays my toned arms are celebrated! It just goes to show

that we should never allow current fashions to determine the state of our health and fitness.

Even though it's probably not part of your job description to be in excellent shape, it is very likely a desire of yours. No matter your size or the label you've given your body, know that most women deal with insecurities. Some of you want to lose weight, some want to gain weight, and still others want more definition. What do we all have in common? We're all striving to feel great in our own skin.

Every minute you exercise contributes to a healthy, strong, toned, and beautiful body. On top of that, exercising makes you feel fantastic! Well, maybe not at the very beginning of the workout—but when you are drenched in sweat and endorphins are rushing through your body at the end of it, you feel good about yourself, right? Still, even though you know how awesome it makes you feel, you might not exercise consistently or as often as you would like. And you are not alone! Most of my clients find it challenging. The three most common mental obstacles to consistent exercise are listed below. Let's see if I can help you turn these obstacles into opportunities by giving you a new perspective.

EXCUSE 1:

"I don't have enough time to exercise."

Why do other people have time to exercise? Because they make time. We all get twenty-four hours in a day and seven days in a week. Every week we have a total of 168 hours to do everything we need to do: work, eat, sleep, etc. What if I asked you to dedicate as little as 1.8 percent of those 168 hours to exercising? Sounds like a tiny time investment, right? Because it is! It's only three 1-hour or six 30-minute sweat sessions. Do you still not have time to exercise?

EXCUSE 2:

"I don't have money for a gym membership."

You don't need a gym membership. You barely need any money to exercise. All you need is a pair of supportive sneakers and some comfy clothes, and off you go. There are many great exercise programs you can download online and countless free YouTube videos available, all with twenty-four-hour access. And let's not forget the great outdoors; you can always go for a run, hike, or bike ride if weather permits. There are so many exercise options for little or no cost! What you really need is commitment. How committed to better health are you?

EXCUSE 3:

"I don't know where to start. I'm so out of shape!"

A group class might feel a bit intimidating, a 3-mile run is out of the question, and even though there are lots of other options, nothing really appeals to you. No worries—it happens! Start with a 5-minute jog, then 10 lunges, 10 squats, and 5 push-ups. Anything that gets you moving! Create your own fun little routine and stick to it for a week or two. When you feel ready, go for a 10-minute jog, do 20 lunges, 20 squats, and 10 push-ups. Before you know it, you've increased your efforts by 100 percent. That's a good feeling, right?

Make exercise nonnegotiable; make it as important as a work appointment! Schedule it and stick to it. Through exercising frequently, you'll build another muscle called "discipline," and this will help you tremendously in other areas of your life. You can do this!

CHEMICALS

Isn't it crazy to think that some of your favorite food items might be laden with toxic chemicals?

Why would a brand you trust put chemicals that can make you sick in their products? Unfortunately, for the majority of companies, it's all about money, not your health. In order to sell more product, food manufacturers use thousands of laboratory-created additives to make our food appear fresher and more attractive or last longer on the shelf.

Certain chemicals in our food disrupt the function of our hormones and create an imbalance of good and bad bacteria in our gut. And some of these additives can even encourage the body to hang on to excess fat! It's important to read labels; be especially wary of ingredients that are hard to pronounce. If you are unsure what an ingredient is, search online to check if it might be harmful to your well-being.

Be aware that toxic chemicals are not just found in the food you're eating. There's a good chance that your cosmetic products, like body lotion, toothpaste, body wash, and facial cleanser, contain harmful chemicals, too. And even though you don't ingest them, they do get absorbed into the bloodstream through your skin and can affect your body and brain.

We rarely think about caring for our brains, but they're fundamentally involved in everything we do. When your brain is healthy and is working right, you are going to feel so much better than when your brain is compromised. And in the end, it's all about feeling great, right? We are all looking to be happy, and taking excellent care of your body and mind is certainly one of the best long-term investments you can make for lasting happiness.

Just changing your eating habits and eliminating processed foods and toxic beauty products from your life will give your brain and body the opportunity to function properly. Fortunately, more companies than ever before are producing great health products. Look for the ones with the fewest ingredients, and aim for labels that include words like "all natural," "organic," "non-GMO," "grass-fed," and "sprouted." A health food store might feel a little intimidating at first, but that will quickly pass when you discover that you don't have to give up your favorite foods—you are just getting better versions of them.

Go explore, have fun with it, and think quality over quantity. You deserve the very best!

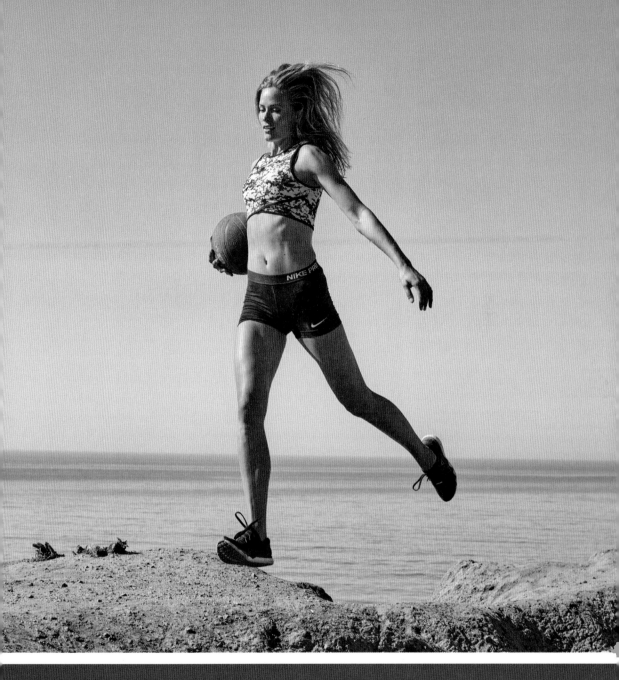

WORK OUT BECAUSE YOU LOVE YOUR BODY
NOT BECAUSE YOU HATE IT

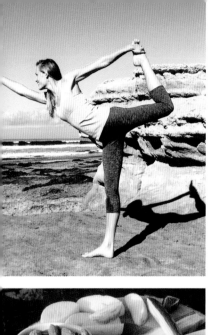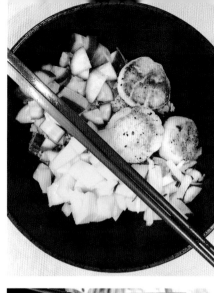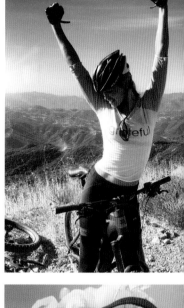
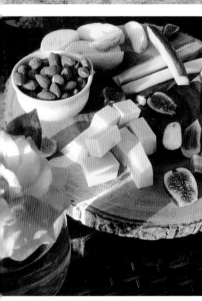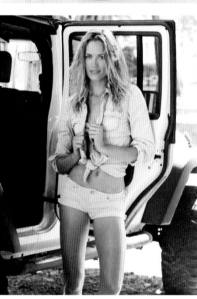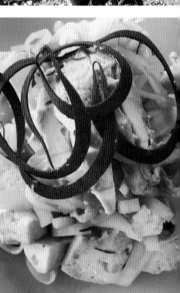
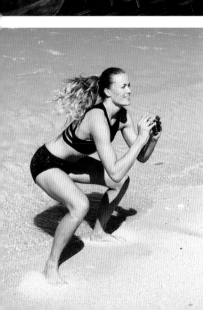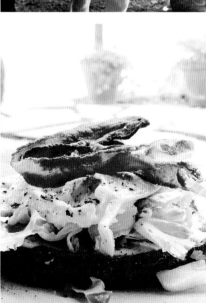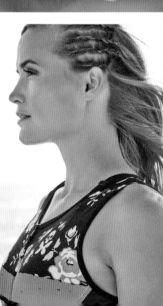

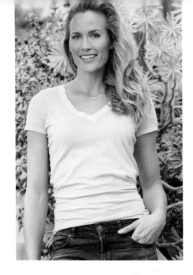

Protein Power

JILL DE JONG

When I started modeling at age seventeen, I was introduced to calorie counting. I thought that it was part of my job to keep track of them and I made a game of it; I tried to eat as much as I could with the least amount of calories.

It took up so much headspace. I was snacking all day, consuming diet products, and skipping meals. I felt hungry all the time. No fun! After several years, I was fed up with feeling deprived. I wanted to eat without feeling guilty or scared and to enjoy food like I used to. It was time to educate myself about food and nutrition to help me understand what I should eat and what I should avoid.

I started listening to my body again, asking what it needed instead of basing every choice on calorie counts. Learning how to cook has helped me tremendously in this process.

NATIONALITY: Dutch

LIVES IN: Los Angeles, CA, USA

CERTIFICATIONS: Institute for Integrative Nutrition Health Coach, AFAA personal trainer, triathlon coach, Matthew Kenney Raw Food Certification

FAVORITE WAYS TO MOVE: High-intensity interval training (HIIT), running, cycling, yoga

KITCHEN MUST-HAVES: Vitamix, sharp knives, cumin, fresh basil, truffle oil, salt

SEEN IN/KNOWN FOR: Peloton, *Fitness*, *Women's Health*, Escada perfume, L'Oréal, Avon, Izod, represented Lara Croft (the Angel of Darkness)

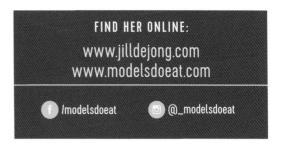

FIND HER ONLINE:
www.jilldejong.com
www.modelsdoeat.com

f /modelsdoeat @_modelsdoeat

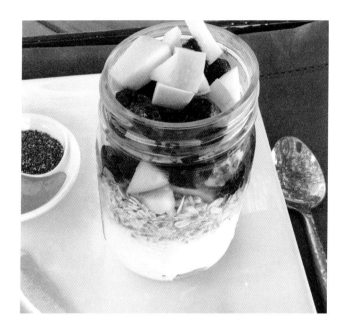

BREAKFAST ON THE GO

If you get up early and don't have an appetite yet or you prefer five minutes' extra sleep over preparing breakfast, then you should try this deliciously simple yogurt treat. Make it the night before, stick it in the fridge, and bring it to work the next day. If you start the day with a jar filled with goodness, it will be much easier to say no to the bagels, croissants, and donuts that will try to seduce you along the way.

INGREDIENTS (1 Serving):

1 cup Greek yogurt
½ cup freshly squeezed orange juice
Raw honey, to taste
½ cup rolled oats
2 tablespoons sunflower seeds, unsalted
1 tablespoon chia seeds (optional)
Your choice of chopped fruit

DIRECTIONS:

1. Place the yogurt in a mason jar.
2. Add the juice, sweeten the mixture with a little raw honey, and stir until smooth.
3. Add the oats, sunflower seeds, chia seeds (if using), and your choice of fruit. Stir to combine.
4. Cover the jar and store in the refrigerator for up to 3 days.

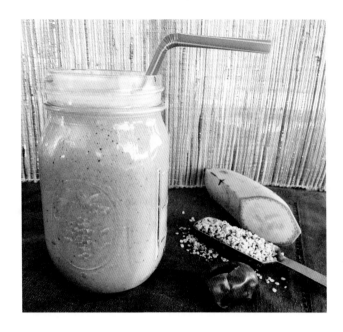

CHOCOLATY PROTEIN SHAKE

I have yet to meet someone who doesn't like a yummy chocolate shake. No wonder there are so many premade protein shakes on the market! But most of them have tons of sugar, or worse, toxic artificial sweeteners. I like to use dates, a nutritious whole food sweetener. This is a great post-workout shake.

INGREDIENTS (1 Serving):

½ cup ice

1 banana

1 cup soy or nut milk

2 tablespoons hemp seeds

1 tablespoon organic peanut butter

1 tablespoon raw cacao

1 Medjool date, pitted

Splash pure vanilla extract

DIRECTIONS:

1. Place all the ingredients in a powerful blender and blend until smooth, then enjoy!

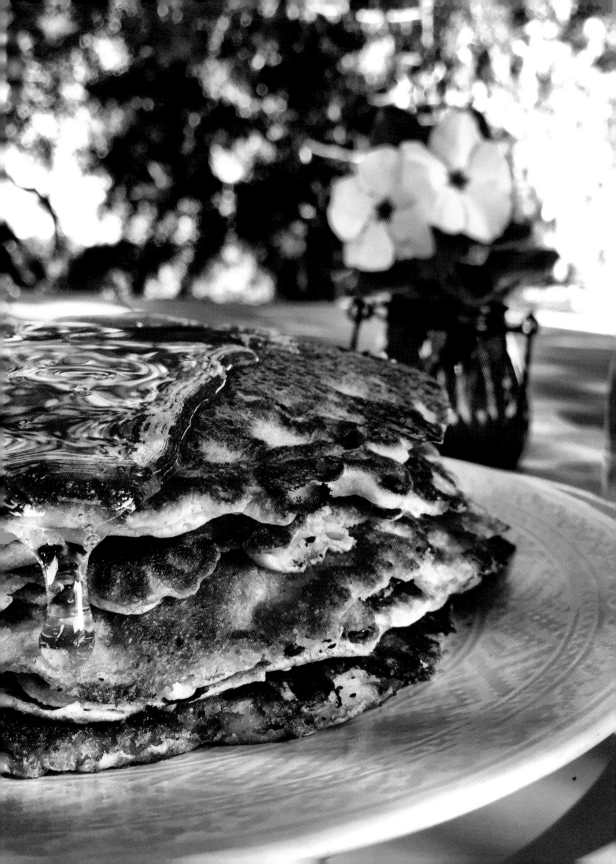

POWER PANCAKES

My parents used to make pancakes for dinner, so it never occurred to me it was a breakfast option until I moved to the States. I think you'll agree that pancakes are delicious any time of the day, hot or cold, thin or thick, rolled or cut up. I like to make more than I can eat so I have a few to snack on the next day. These nutritious protein-packed power pancakes will make any day feel like a Sunday.

INGREDIENTS (2–3 Servings):

⅓ cup oat flour (or rolled oats finely ground in a food processor)

¼ cup rolled oats

1 teaspoon baking powder

½ teaspoon baking soda

⅓ cup cottage cheese

3 organic pasture-raised eggs, lightly beaten

3 tablespoons milk (dairy or plant-based)

1 teaspoon extra-virgin olive oil, plus more for the pan

1 teaspoon pure vanilla extract

Pinch of salt

Optional toppings: unsweetened shredded coconut, raw honey, butter, banana

DIRECTIONS:

1. In a medium bowl, mix the oat flour, rolled oats, baking powder, and baking soda together.

2. Add the cottage cheese, eggs, milk, olive oil, vanilla, and salt and whisk just until smooth. You should still see cottage cheese and oats floating in the batter. (Alternatively, pulse the mixture in a blender until just combined.)

3. Heat a frying pan over medium-high heat, add a little olive oil to the pan, and coat the pan evenly.

4. Pour ¼ cup of batter into the hot pan and cook until the edges of the pancake start to dry and bubbles begin forming in the middle. Flip and cook for another minute.

5. Transfer the pancake to a plate and cover or place it in a warm oven while you prepare the rest.

6. Top with your favorite toppings and enjoy!

"I set fitness goals to stay focused. Exercise helps me develop two important muscles: willpower and discipline. Those muscles are of great use in all areas of life. I love getting out of my comfort zone over and over again!"

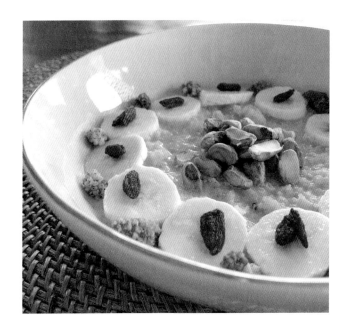

EXOTIC QUINOA BREAKFAST BOWL

Quinoa for breakfast might sound a little strange at first. But this flavorful and nourishing breakfast bowl is going to win you over. It's easy to digest and will give you lots of energy for the day ahead.

Want to save time in the morning? On Sunday, make a big pot of quinoa for the week. This recipe will only take 5 minutes to make when the quinoa is already cooked.

INGREDIENTS (1 Serving):

1 cup cooked quinoa
½–¾ cup almond milk or your milk of choice
1 teaspoon extra-virgin coconut oil
Pinch of salt

TOPPINGS

½ banana, sliced
2 tablespoons goji berries
1 handful dried mulberries
1 handful pistachios
Pure maple syrup (optional)

DIRECTIONS:

1. Put the quinoa and almond milk in a small pan, and stir in the coconut oil and salt.
2. Cook over medium-high heat for 3 to 4 minutes, or until heated through.
3. Transfer to a bowl and add the toppings. Drizzle with a little maple syrup, if desired.

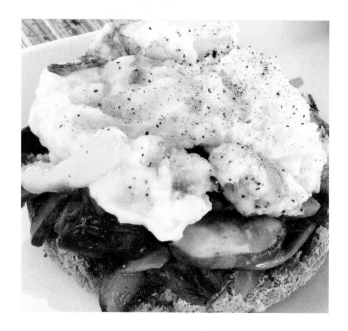

VEGAN MORNING SCRAMBLE

I can eat breakfast all day. With so many healthy choices, I hardly ever eat the same breakfast two days in a row. When I wake up and crave something savory and light, I eat this yummy scramble. And if I have a bigger appetite, I'll add a slice of toasted bread.

INGREDIENTS (1 Serving):

1–2 teaspoons extra-virgin olive oil
1 cup spinach
3–4 ounces cubed tofu
½ cup finely chopped leek
1 teaspoon soy sauce

DIRECTIONS:

1. Heat the olive oil in a medium skillet over medium-high heat.
2. Stir-fry the spinach, tofu, and leek for 3 to 5 minutes, until the leek softens and the spinach wilts. Stir in the soy sauce.
3. Transfer to a plate and serve.

CARROT QUINOA BOWL

We've become a quinoa-eating nation! And I get why; it's a versatile superfood, gluten-free, and one of the few vegetarian "complete" proteins. I personally find plain quinoa a bit boring and usually make it with chicken or veggie stock to add flavor. But this recipe goes beyond that, adding an exotic touch to the meal by combining fresh carrot juice with nourishing ginger and onion.

INGREDIENTS (2 Servings):

QUINOA

2 teaspoons extra-virgin olive oil
½ cup finely chopped yellow onion
1½ cups fresh carrot juice
½ tablespoon finely grated ginger
1 cup quinoa, rinsed well

TOPPINGS

½ cup sliced almonds
⅔ cup chopped apple
½ avocado, sliced or chopped
2 tablespoons shredded unsweetened coconut
Sea salt, to taste

DIRECTIONS:

1. Heat a saucepan over medium-high heat. Add the olive oil and onion and sauté until translucent, about 3 minutes.
2. Stir in the carrot juice, ginger, and quinoa.
3. Bring to a boil and reduce the heat to low. Cover and simmer until all the liquid is absorbed, 15 to 20 minutes.
4. Let rest, covered, for 5 minutes, then fluff with a fork.
5. While the quinoa is simmering, lightly toast the almonds in a dry sauté pan.
6. Divide the quinoa and toppings between two plates. Season slightly with salt to enhance sweetness, and serve.

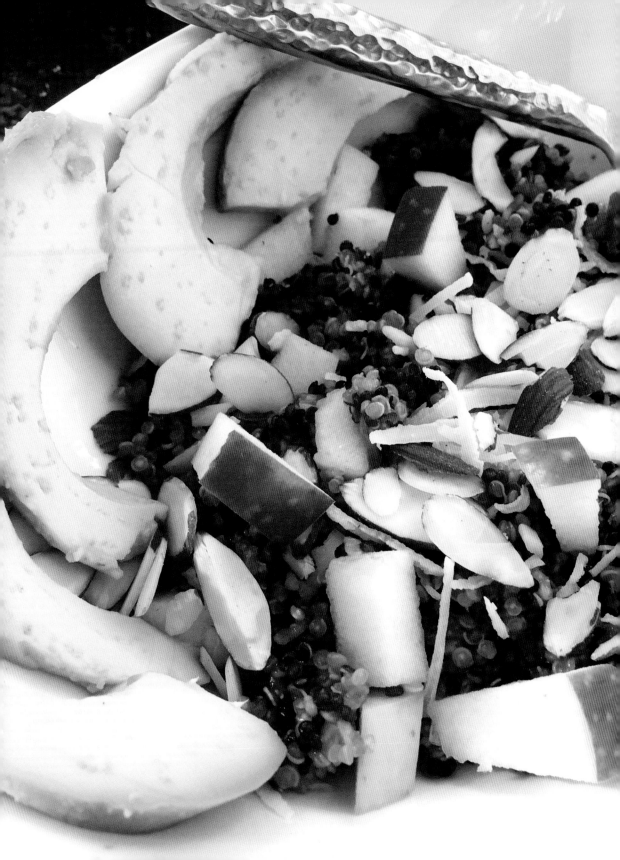

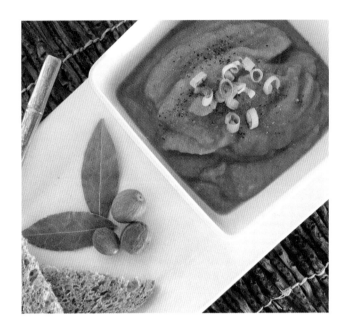

EASY PEA-SY SOUP

Want an easy way to eat more veggies? Make a soup! After a bowl of this very-easy-to-make split pea soup, I feel satisfied and full for hours. You can't go wrong including split peas in your diet, as they are highly nutritious and rich in protein.

INGREDIENTS (4 Servings):

7 cups vegetable broth

2 cups dried green split peas, picked over and rinsed well

1½ cups chopped yellow onion

1 cup chopped carrot

2 garlic cloves, minced

¼ teaspoon ground cumin

½ teaspoon sea salt, plus more to taste

¼ teaspoon freshly ground black pepper

2 bay leaves

Pinch of nutmeg

Optional toppings: shredded carrots, sliced scallions

DIRECTIONS:

1. In a large pan or Dutch oven, combine all the ingredients and bring to a boil over high heat.
2. Reduce the heat, cover, and simmer for 1 hour, or until the peas are tender, stirring occasionally.
3. Remove the bay leaves and blend the soup until smooth using an immersion (stick) or traditional blender, then transfer back to the pan. Thin with water or more broth if desired.
4. Garnish with shredded carrots and scallions (if using), and add more salt to taste.

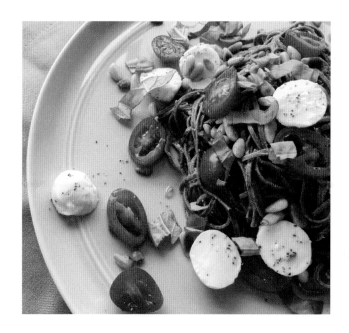

BLACK BEAN PESTO PASTA

Black bean noodles are a pasta lover's dream; their muscle-building protein, belly-filling fiber, and energizing nutrients will make you throw out all their nutritionally deficient white-flour siblings. Eating pasta has never felt this good!

INGREDIENTS (2 Servings):

1 (8-ounce) package black bean spaghetti
¼ cup pesto (store-bought or homemade)
1 cup cherry tomatoes, halved
½ cup diced fresh mozzarella
⅓ cup chopped fresh basil
¼ cup toasted pine nuts
Sea salt and freshly ground black pepper, to taste

DIRECTIONS:

1. Cook the spaghetti according to package directions, then drain.
2. Return the spaghetti to the pot and add the pesto. Stir to coat thoroughly.
3. Divide the pasta between two serving bowls and top with the tomatoes, mozzarella, basil, and pine nuts. Season with salt and pepper and serve immediately.

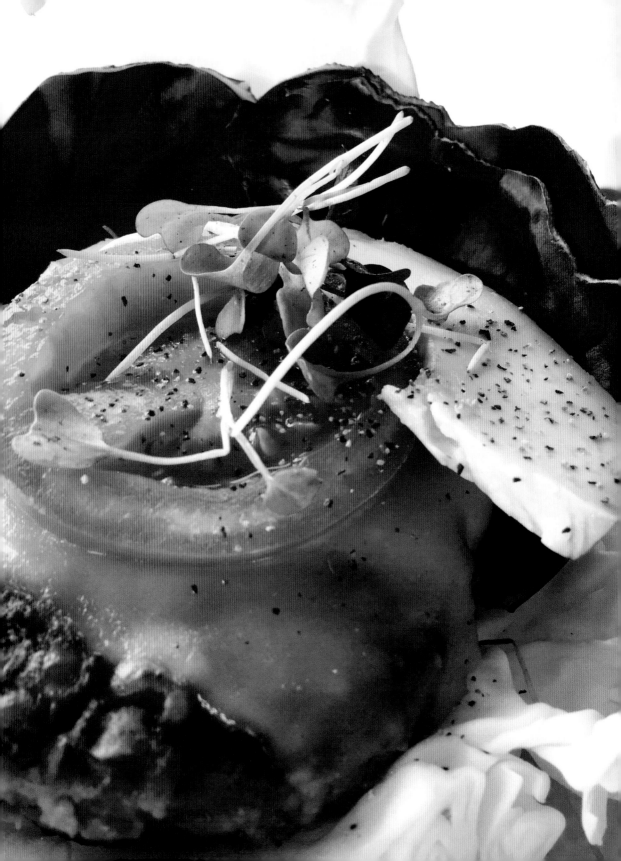

GARBANZO TRUFFLE BURGER

Why eat an ordinary burger when you can eat an extraordinary one? The decadent flavor of truffle oil combined with cheese is to die for! And only a third of this burger is made with beef. Less meat plus more nutrition and flavor sounds almost too good to be true, right? And yet here it is. As with any recipe, always aim for the highest-quality ingredients—in this case, organic, grass-fed beef.

INGREDIENTS (1 Serving):

¼ cup canned chickpeas, rinsed and drained

¼ cup chopped yellow onion

¼ cup ground beef

Sea salt and freshly ground black pepper, to taste

¼ teaspoon truffle oil

1 tablespoon extra-virgin olive oil

2 slices Gouda or cheddar cheese (optional)

Bibb or other sturdy lettuce, for serving

Optional toppings: avocado, tomato

DIRECTIONS:

1. In a mixing bowl, mash the chickpeas with a fork, then add the onion and beef. Combine thoroughly.

2. Season with salt and pepper to taste and mix in the truffle oil.

3. Knead the mixture well, then form into a ball. Press into a burger shape, making sure the edges are solid and rounded.

4. Heat the olive oil in a skillet over medium-high heat. Place the burger in the skillet and cook, turning once, until browned on both sides and cooked through, 3 to 5 minutes each side.

5. Top the burger with cheese (if using) and let melt.

6. To serve, wrap the burger in a piece of lettuce with your favorite toppings (or serve on a salad) and enjoy!

LENTILS WITH SALMON AND BROCCOLI

This truly is a power protein team! A 3-ounce piece of salmon and 1 cup of cooked lentils add up to 35 grams of protein. I'm a big fan of lots of cumin in my lentils to add warm, nutty flavor notes to the dish. This recipe makes more lentils than you need, so you can whip up a big batch, then enjoy more over the next few days. Try lentils for breakfast with an egg, or add a little broth for a quick soup.

INGREDIENTS (2 Servings):

LENTILS (6–8 Servings)

2–3 tablespoons extra-virgin olive oil

1 medium yellow onion, chopped

2 large carrots, chopped

1 medium zucchini, chopped

1 teaspoon ground cumin

1 teaspoon sea salt, plus more to taste

1 quart chicken or vegetable stock

2 bay leaves (optional)

1 (16-ounce) bag organic lentils, picked over and rinsed well

SALMON

2 (3-ounce) center-cut salmon fillets

Sea salt and freshly ground black pepper

2 tablespoons extra-virgin olive oil

BROCCOLI

2 heads broccoli, chopped into florets

Lemon wedges, for serving

DIRECTIONS:

LENTILS

1. Heat the olive oil in a medium pot. Stir in the onion, carrots, and zucchini.
2. Sauté over medium-high heat until the veggies are slightly soft, about 5 minutes.
3. Season with cumin and salt, then add the stock and bay leaves (if using).
4. Add the lentils, bring to a boil, and reduce the heat to low.
5. Simmer for 45 to 60 minutes, or until the lentils are soft. Remove the bay leaves before serving.

SALMON

1. Season the fish all over with salt and pepper.
2. Warm the olive oil in a large nonstick skillet over medium heat.
3. Raise the heat to medium-high, then place the salmon in the pan, skin side up. Cook until golden brown, about 4 minutes.
4. Turn the fish over with a spatula, and cook until it feels firm to the touch, about 3 minutes more.

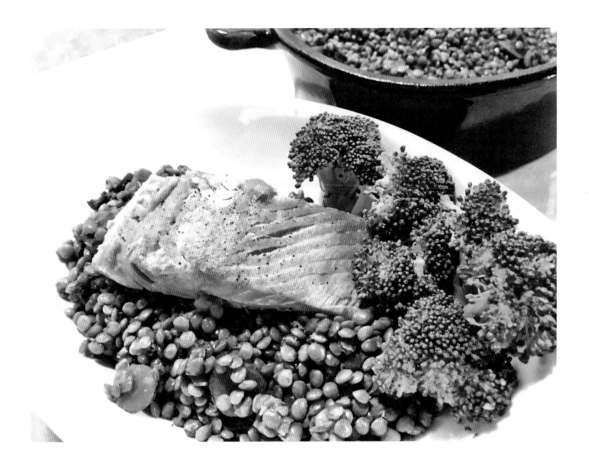

BROCCOLI

1. Bring a large pot of water to a rapid boil, and prepare a bowl of ice water.
2. Add the broccoli to the pot and cook until crisp-tender, 2 to 4 minutes.
3. Remove with a slotted spoon and plunge immediately into the ice water, then drain.
4. Divide one-third of the lentils between two plates, reserving the rest for leftovers, then top with the salmon and broccoli and serve immediately with a wedge of lemon.

SCRUMPTIOUS SCALLOPS

Looking for a great alternative to red meat? Look no further! Scallops are the perfect lean protein choice. They are surprisingly easy to make, and even friends who don't like fish will likely enjoy eating this delicious dish. Scallops have a mild seafood flavor and smooth, buttery texture. Pair with sautéed kale and roasted sweet potatoes or serve over a bed of salad.

INGREDIENTS (1 Serving):

3 ounces sea scallops
Sea salt and freshly ground black pepper, to taste
2 tablespoons extra-virgin olive oil
Lemon wedges, for serving (optional)

DIRECTIONS:

1. Gently pat the scallops with a paper towel until completely dry, then season with salt and pepper.
2. Heat the olive oil in a nonstick skillet over high heat.
3. Add the scallops, flat side down, and let cook without touching them until they are well browned, about 2 minutes.
4. Flip the scallops to sear on the other side for another 1 to 2 minutes, depending on size and thickness, taking care not to overcook.
5. Serve immediately, dressed with a squeeze of lemon, if desired.

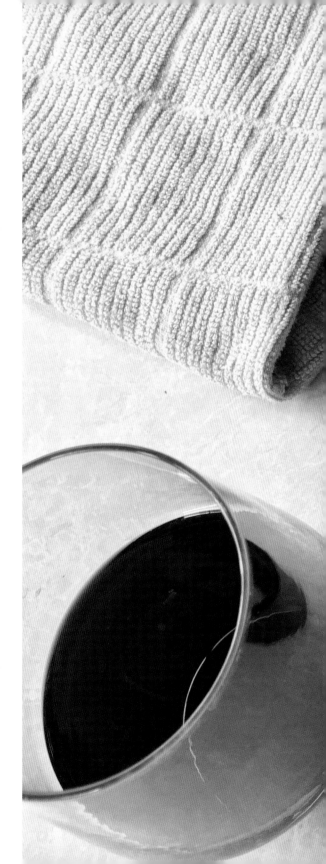

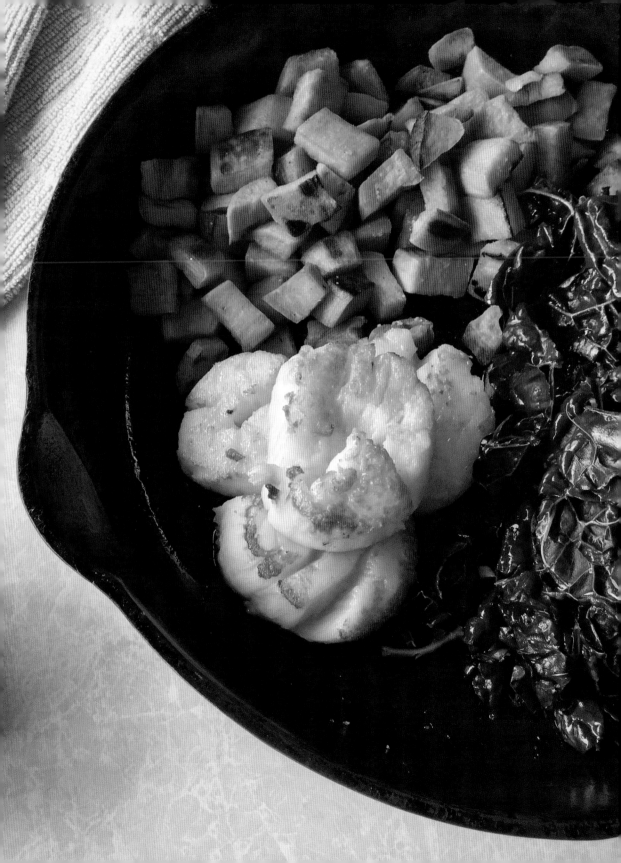

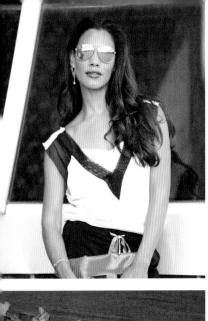
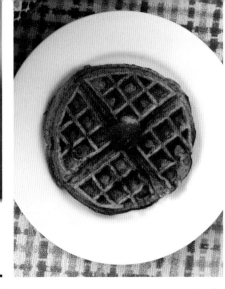
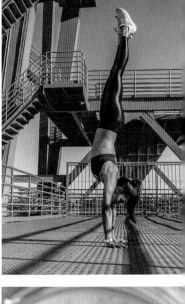
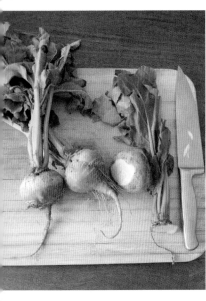
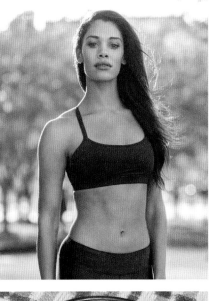
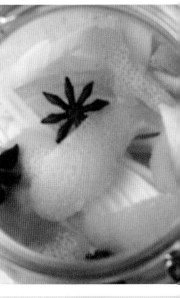
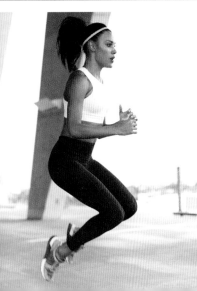
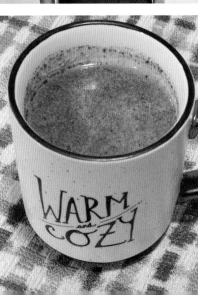
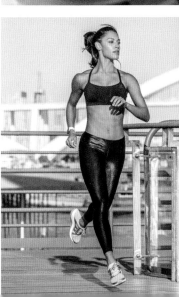

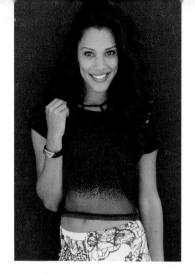

Less Sugar, More Spice

TAYLOR WALKER SINNING

One of my biggest struggles has been learning not to judge myself with regard to my body. I have learned to embrace my strong quads and thighs, which allowed me years of passionate dancing, and my (sometimes bloated) belly, which has allowed me to enjoy delicious meals with people I love. I am honestly so grateful for the skin I am in.

The shift from food to satisfy to food as fuel happened only a few short years ago. Once I moved out of my childhood home, I started playing with fresh flavors and spices and cut out most packaged foods. Much to my surprise, my palate changed within weeks! Fruits tasted sweeter. My dessert cravings were satiated with melon or a yogurt parfait. I also learned that a little salt and lots of spice go a long way. My spice cabinet runneth over, and my meals never taste bland.

NATIONALITY: American

LIVES IN: Miami, FL, USA

DEGREES/CERTIFICATIONS: Nutritious Life Certified, CPT, pre/postnatal corrective exercise specialist, M.S. in K–12 physical education, Spartan SGX

FAVORITE WAYS TO MOVE: Tabata, boot camp, barre, yoga, kickboxing

KITCHEN MUST-HAVES: NutriBullet for making soups, sauces, and smoothies, and red pepper and hot sauce for spicing things up. I love heat!

SEEN IN/KNOWN FOR: Under Armour, Nike, Peloton, *Fitness*, *Shape*, Champions, HSN, Target, Goya

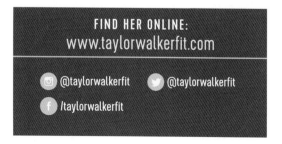

FIND HER ONLINE:
www.taylorwalkerfit.com

@taylorwalkerfit   @taylorwalkerfit
/taylorwalkerfit

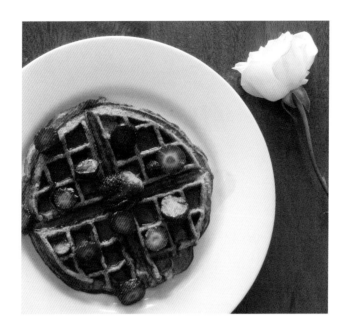

FLOURLESS FLAX WAFFLE

Pancakes and waffles are my favorite indulgences, but the sugar crash that comes with them is not. I created this recipe as a great pre- or post-workout treat that is not only filling, but also satisfying and comforting at once. The sweetness from ripe bananas helps caramelize the waffle, and not only do they freeze well, but you can also make the batter days in advance and throw it in the waffle iron straight from the refrigerator for an easy weekend breakfast.

INGREDIENTS (1–2 Servings):

2 organic pasture-raised eggs
1 teaspoon ground cinnamon
2 tablespoons ground flaxseed
½ teaspoon pure vanilla extract
1 ripe banana, mashed
Cooking spray

DIRECTIONS:

1. Preheat a waffle iron and set to Level 6.
2. Combine all the ingredients in a bowl and whisk until smooth.
3. Lightly coat the iron with cooking spray and fill with batter.
4. Cook for about 5 minutes, then serve with your favorite toppings.

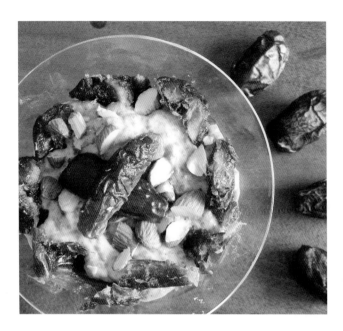

CHIA BANANA PARFAIT

This recipe will yield enough pudding for the entire week, so I usually make it on Sunday night. It's a great pre-workout breakfast to help you get the most out of your sweat session, the natural way.

INGREDIENTS (7 Servings):

1 ripe banana

1 (13.5-ounce) can low-fat coconut milk

1 teaspoon ground cinnamon

1 teaspoon pure vanilla extract

¼ cup chia seeds

½ teaspoon extra-virgin coconut oil

2 tablespoons roughly chopped almonds

1 Medjool date, pitted and chopped

Raw honey (optional)

DIRECTIONS:

1. In a blender, combine the banana, coconut milk, cinnamon, and vanilla and blend until smooth, then transfer to a bowl.

2. Whisk in the chia seeds, cover, and let stand in the refrigerator for 2 to 3 hours, until the mixture thickens into a pudding.

3. While the pudding chills, melt the coconut oil in a skillet over medium-low heat. Add the almonds and toast until crispy, stirring often and taking care not to let them burn.

4. In a glass or bowl, layer in order: pudding, chopped date, almonds, and a drizzle of honey (if using).

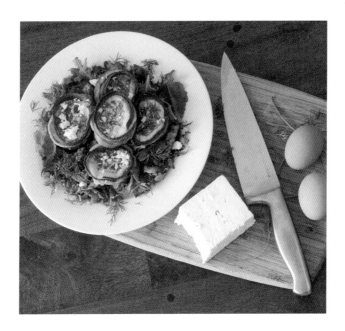

MEDITERRANEAN BREAKFAST CUPS

The egg is one of the most versatile health foods out there. I made the switch to free-range, organic eggs a couple of years back, and what a difference it has made! The Mediterranean flavors in this recipe are fresh, and these cups are easy to make ahead of time. A quick trip to the microwave, and you have an on-the-go, protein-packed breakfast that will make you scream "Opa!" with every bite.

INGREDIENTS (4 Servings):

Cooking spray

8 slices turkey bacon (optional)

5 organic pasture-raised eggs plus 2 egg whites, beaten

2 tablespoons plain Greek yogurt

5–6 banana pepper rings or black olives, chopped

¼ cup seeded and chopped tomato

Freshly ground black pepper

2 tablespoons crumbled feta cheese, for serving

2 tablespoons roughly chopped fresh dill, for serving

DIRECTIONS:

1. Preheat the oven to 350°F.
2. Lightly coat 8 cups of a standard muffin tin with cooking spray, then line the cups with one slice of turkey bacon each (if using).
3. Gently combine the eggs, yogurt, peppers or olives, and tomato in a bowl, then season with a few grinds of black pepper.
4. Fill each cup halfway with the egg mixture and bake for 30 to 35 minutes, or until thoroughly cooked.
5. Garnish with the crumbled feta and fresh dill.

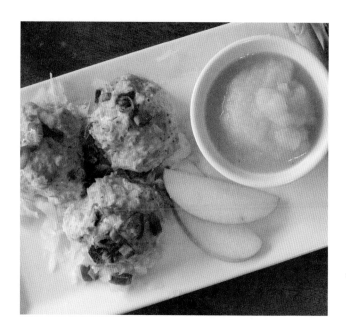

SWEET AND SAVORY CHICKEN MEATBALLS

Sweet and savory is the name of my cooking game. These meatballs are light and fluffy, and use quinoa and egg as binding agents instead of breadcrumbs. This keeps the gluten to a minimum while amping up the protein factor! Eat them alone, on a sandwich, or served with sauerkraut and applesauce. Just one batch will give you versatile lunches all week.

INGREDIENTS (6 Servings):

1 pound ground chicken

½ cup cooked quinoa

1 egg, beaten

2 celery stalks, chopped

4 Medjool dates, pitted and chopped

2 tablespoons whipped cream cheese

1 tablespoon whole-grain mustard

1 teaspoon chopped fresh sage

1 teaspoon celery seed

Cooking spray

2 scallions, chopped, for garnish

DIRECTIONS:

1. Preheat the oven to 350°F.
2. Combine the chicken, quinoa, egg, celery, dates, cream cheese, mustard, sage, and celery seed in a bowl and mix well. Form into 2-inch meatballs.
3. Spray a baking sheet or mini-muffin tin with cooking spray and arrange the meatballs so that they are not touching.
4. Bake for 15 minutes, or until firm to the touch. Garnish with chopped scallions.

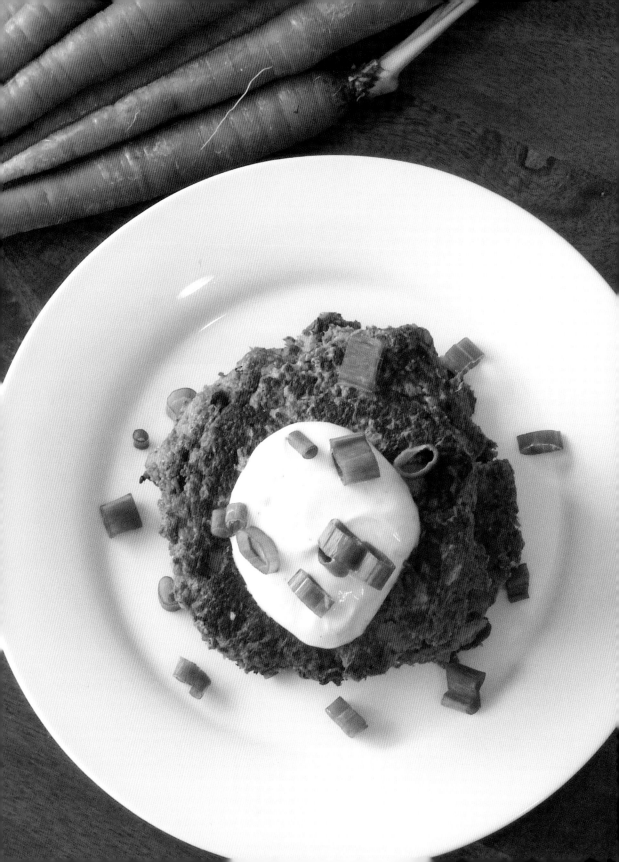

SWEET POTATO CAKES

Light and fluffy, these sweet potato cakes are a great alternative to traditional potato latkes. I like to top mine with a sunny-side-up or poached egg and some sliced scallion. You can also add them to a salad or eat them as a side. The maple dipping sauce is a must-try!

INGREDIENTS (4 Servings):

SWEET POTATO CAKES

1 sweet potato, baked, peeled, and mashed
¼ cup ground flaxseed
1 large egg, beaten
1 tablespoon pure maple syrup
2 teaspoons ground cinnamon
1 teaspoon ground nutmeg
1 teaspoon ground turmeric
1–2 tablespoons extra-virgin coconut oil, for frying
2 scallions, chopped, for garnish

DIPPING SAUCE

2 tablespoons Greek yogurt
1 tablespoon pure maple syrup
4–5 dashes hot sauce, to taste

DIRECTIONS:

SWEET POTATO CAKES

1. Combine the potato, flaxseed, egg, maple syrup, cinnamon, nutmeg, and turmeric in a mixing bowl, stirring well to combine thoroughly.
2. Heat the coconut oil in a skillet over medium-high heat.
3. Form the mixture into four 4-inch patties and cook like pancakes, turning once, until lightly browned and very crisp, about 3 minutes per side.
4. Garnish with scallions and serve immediately with the dipping sauce.

DIPPING SAUCE

1. Whisk together the Greek yogurt and maple syrup, then season to taste with hot sauce.

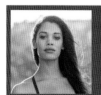

"These days, cooking is my 'yoga,' so to speak. There is no greater joy than cooking for people I love. I try my best to be healthy during the week, and I let myself indulge on the weekends. Not every meal, but definitely one or two. This helps me stay on the straight and narrow during the week!"

SOUTHWESTERN BLACK BEAN BURGER

This recipe reminds me of my journey to health and fitness. I needed something healthy at a concert, and they offered me a black bean burger. To my surprise, I loved it and realized that healthy food could also be delicious! Dense, filling, and full of fiber, this burger features flavors that will take you south of the border. Adjust the amount of cayenne to make this as spicy (or not) as you like. The patties can be frozen for later and quickly heated on the stovetop in a little coconut oil. Serve hot over a taco salad, on a bun, or just wrapped in sturdy lettuce.

INGREDIENTS (4 Servings):

1 (15-ounce) can black beans, rinsed and drained
½ red bell pepper, finely chopped
½ white or yellow onion, finely chopped
3 garlic cloves, crushed
1 scallion, thinly sliced
1 handful fresh cilantro, chopped
1 egg, beaten
½ cup oat flour (or rolled oats finely ground in food processor)
1–3 teaspoons cayenne
1 teaspoon sweet paprika
1 teaspoon hot sauce
¼ cup coconut flour, for coating
1 tablespoon extra-virgin olive or coconut oil
Whole wheat buns (optional, for serving)

DIRECTIONS:

1. In a mixing bowl, mash the black beans into a paste with the tines of a fork.
2. Add the bell pepper, onion, garlic, scallion, cilantro, and egg and mix thoroughly.
3. Slowly fold in the oat flour until the mixture is stuck together and moist.
4. Add the cayenne, paprika, and hot sauce and combine gently until completely mixed.
5. Form 4 patties of equal size and desired thickness and dredge them lightly in the coconut flour.
6. Heat the oil in skillet over medium-high heat and cook each patty for 3 to 5 minutes, turning once, until the egg is set and the patty is firm.
7. Serve immediately on whole wheat buns (if using).

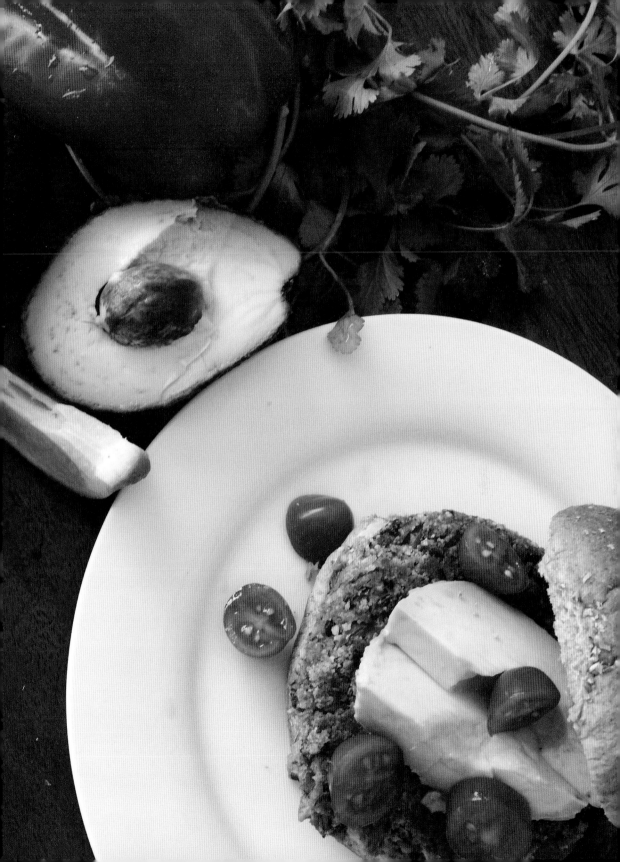

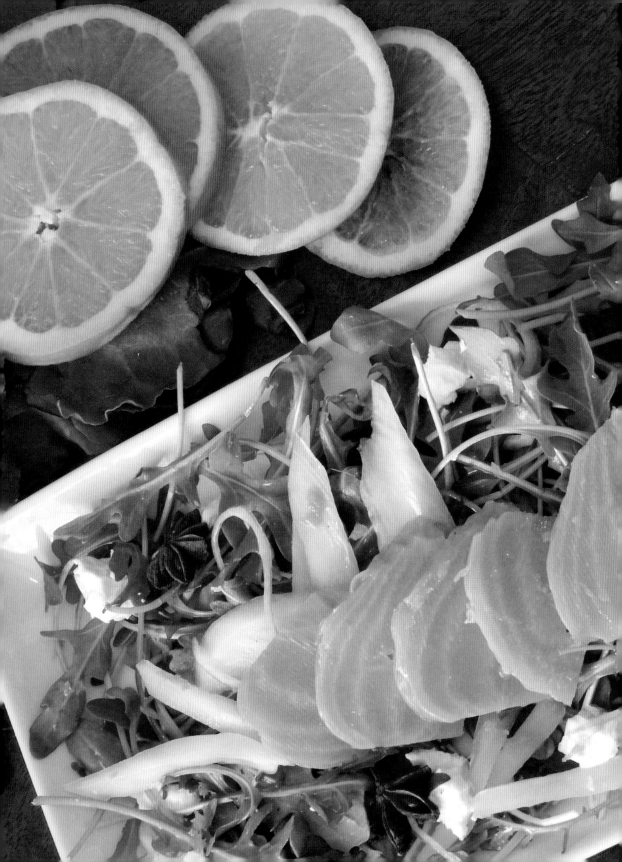

ROASTED BEET SALAD WITH PICKLED FENNEL

Golden beets are less earthy than red and pair beautifully with the tart, citrusy flavor of pickled fennel. Both the beets and the fennel can be made days in advance and stored in the refrigerator. Top this salad with the protein of your choice, like salmon, shrimp, or chicken, and enjoy a light meal with an incredible depth of flavor.

INGREDIENTS (4 Servings):

ROASTED BEETS

1 bunch regular or golden beets, washed, with tops and
  bottoms cut off
1–2 tablespoons extra-virgin olive oil

PICKLED FENNEL

1–2 fennel bulbs
Juice and rind of 1 orange
3–4 star anise pods
2 cups water
1½ cups apple cider vinegar
2 tablespoons sugar
½ teaspoon pickling salt

SALAD

4 cups salad greens of choice
Citrus-infused olive oil (preferably orange)
¼ cup crumbled or sliced goat cheese
White balsamic vinegar
Sea salt and freshly ground black pepper

DIRECTIONS:

ROASTED BEETS

1. Preheat the oven to 400°F.
2. Place the beets on foil and drizzle with the olive oil, then wrap them tightly and place on a baking sheet. Transfer to the oven.
3. Roast for 1 hour, or until the flesh is easily pierced with a fork.
4. Cool completely, then slice thinly and chill until ready to serve.

PICKLED FENNEL

1. Slice the fennel bulbs finely and place them in an airtight jar with the orange rind and the star anise pods.
2. In a small saucepan, bring the water, apple cider vinegar, sugar, salt, and orange juice to a boil over medium-high heat. Cook until the sugar and salt are fully dissolved.
3. Pour the brine over the fennel and let sit for at least 3 hours, but preferably overnight. Store in the refrigerator.

SALAD

1. Toss the greens lightly in citrus olive oil, then top with the fennel (drained), thinly sliced beets, and goat cheese.
2. Dress with 1 part extra citrus olive oil to 3 parts white balsamic vinegar (make as much or as little dressing as you like, and store leftovers in the fridge). Season with a pinch of salt and freshly ground pepper.

PEANUT BUTTER ENERGY BALLS

These simple bites are the perfect on-the-go snack, and you can play with the flavors in endless combinations. They're ready in a flash and a great sweet treat for breakfast or even dessert. Packed with fiber and protein, they'll give you the energy you need to take on the day.

INGREDIENTS (8 Servings):

1 cup quick-cooking rolled oats

1 cup organic peanut butter

½ cup ground flaxseed

⅔ cup slivered almonds

¼ cup raisins

¼ cup raw honey

1 tablespoon chia seeds

1 tablespoon pure vanilla extract

Optional: shredded coconut, chopped dark chocolate, cacao nibs

DIRECTIONS:

1. Mix all the ingredients, in a large bowl until well combined.
2. Break off pieces of the mixture and roll into 1-inch balls.
3. Refrigerate for at least 30 minutes before serving.
4. Store in an airtight container in the refrigerator for up to 10 days.

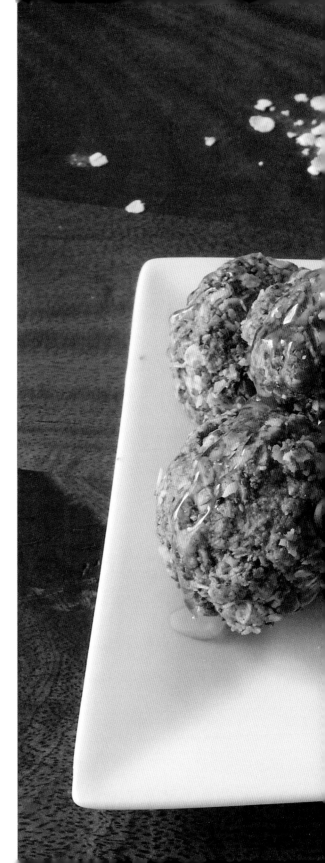

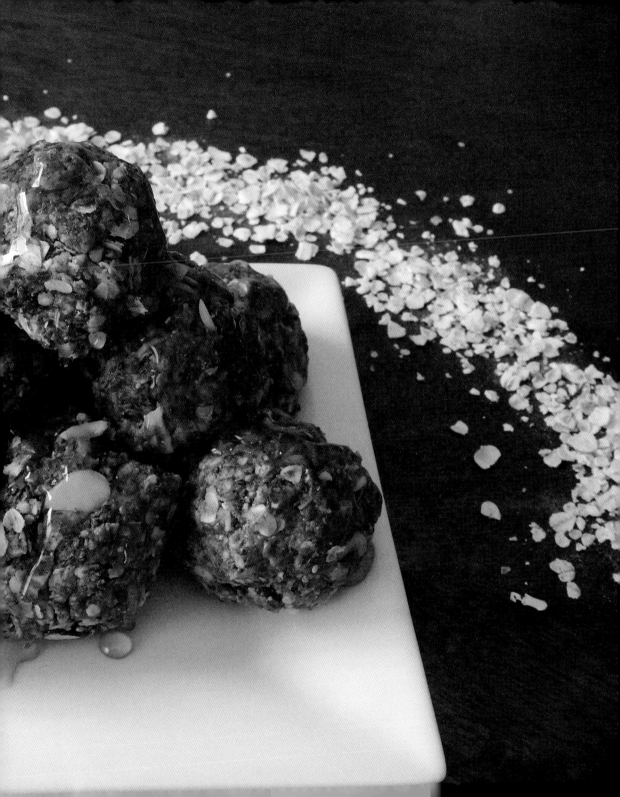

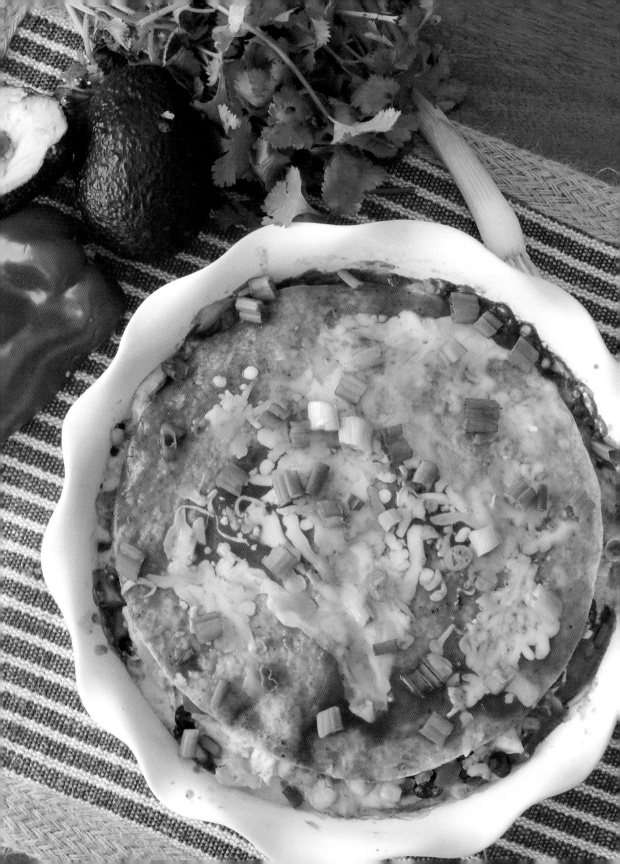

EASY CHICKEN ENCHILADA CASSEROLE

Forget "Taco Tuesday"! This enchilada casserole is an indulgence the entire family will love. You can make this recipe in advance and freeze it for a last-minute weekday dinner, or simply make the filling ahead of time and assemble the casserole when you're ready to bake it. I love to place fresh toppings like salsa, cilantro, and avocado on the table and serve it with a light fruit salad, black beans, and a skinny margarita.

INGREDIENTS (4 Servings):

Cooking spray

1–2 tablespoons extra-virgin olive oil

1 large white onion, diced

1 bell pepper (any color), cored, seeded, and thinly sliced

4 garlic cloves, minced

½ cup mixed black beans and corn (frozen or canned)

2 organic pasture-raised eggs, beaten

½ cup cooked quinoa

1 (12-ounce) can all-natural enchilada sauce

3 (9-inch) whole wheat tortillas

1 rotisserie chicken, shredded (skin and bones discarded), or 2 boneless, skinless chicken breasts, cooked and shredded

½ cup shredded Mexican or cheddar cheese

2 scallions, sliced, for garnish

DIRECTIONS:

1. Preheat the oven to 350°F. Grease a 9-inch pie plate with cooking spray.
2. Heat the olive oil in large skillet over medium-high heat and add the onion, cooking until it begins to soften, 3 to 4 minutes.
3. Add the bell pepper and garlic and cook, stirring constantly, until the color brightens and they begin to soften, 3 to 4 minutes longer.
4. Add the bean and corn mixture and continue to cook until warmed thoroughly. Remove from the heat.
5. In a small bowl, fold the beaten eggs into the quinoa.
6. In the prepared pie plate, layer the enchilada sauce, 1 tortilla, pepper mixture, quinoa mixture, shredded chicken, and a thin layer of cheese. Repeat until all the ingredients are used.
7. Transfer to the oven and bake for 15 to 20 minutes, or until the cheese is melted and bubbly.
8. Cut into wedges, garnish with the scallions, and serve.

GRASS-FED BOLOGNESE SAUCE

My husband and I took a cooking class in Tuscany on our honeymoon and figured out the secret to delicious Italian food: the fresh, organic ingredients they use in all of their dishes. When cooking something indulgent like Bolognese sauce, buy the best grass-fed beef and organic vegetables you can afford. Bolognese is a perfect way to use leftover marinara. Try serving it over spiralized vegetable "pasta" to counterbalance the heavy meat sauce.

INGREDIENTS (4 Servings):

1–2 tablespoons extra-virgin olive oil

1 white onion, chopped

4 garlic cloves, crushed

2 celery stalks, chopped

1–2 carrots, chopped

1 sprig fresh rosemary

1 cup tomato sauce or 1 (14-ounce) can diced tomatoes plus 1 (6-ounce) can tomato paste

¼ cup red wine (optional, or substitute beef or chicken stock)

1 pound grass-fed ground beef

1 teaspoon garlic salt

1–2 teaspoons dried Italian seasoning blend (oregano, basil, parsley)

¼ teaspoon crushed red pepper

Sea salt and freshly ground black pepper, to taste

DIRECTIONS:

1. In a large saucepan, heat the olive oil over medium-high heat. Add the onion and cook until soft, 4 to 5 minutes, then add the garlic, celery, carrot, and rosemary sprig. Cook until almost soft, 5 to 6 minutes, and then remove the rosemary sprig.

2. Add the tomato paste (if using canned diced tomatoes); stir to combine and cook until well blended and thickened, 2 to 3 minutes.

3. Deglaze the pan with the wine or stock and add the ground beef, breaking it up with a wooden spoon to brown evenly.

4. When the meat is mostly browned, add the tomato sauce or diced tomatoes along with the garlic salt, Italian seasoning blend, and crushed red pepper. Bring the mixture to a boil, reduce the heat, and simmer for 15 to 20 minutes.

5. Taste and adjust the spices as needed, then season with salt and pepper.

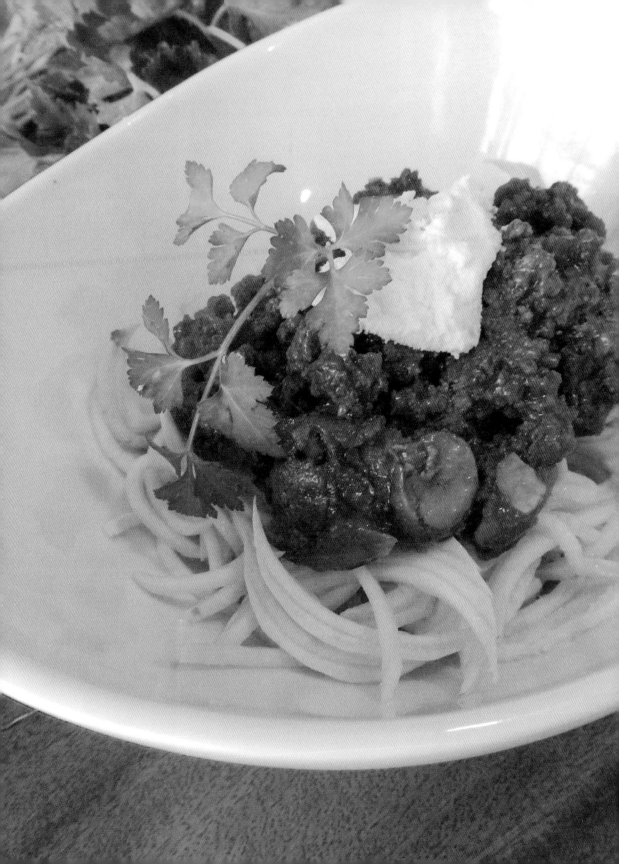

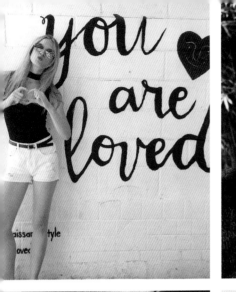
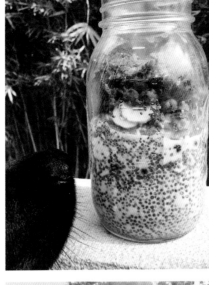
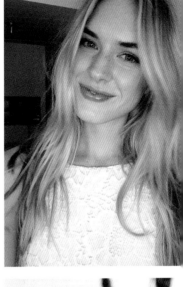
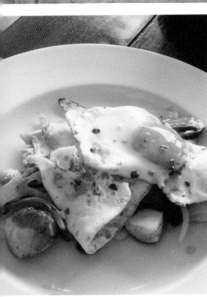
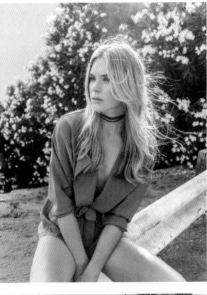
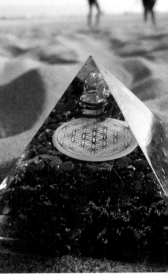
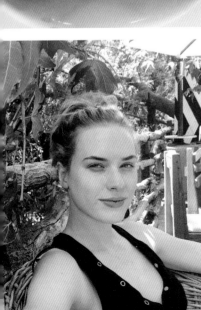
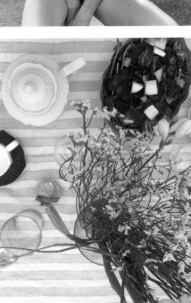
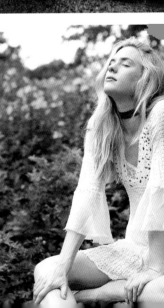

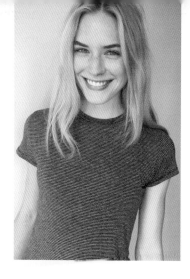

Paleo Party

COURTNEY JAMES

As a young teen, I suffered from stomachaches and a weak immune system. But I ignored the signs my body gave me, which resulted in admissions to hospital—once for appendicitis and once for glandular fever. I realized I had to be more in tune with my body. I took my health into my own hands and learned the ins and outs of what I needed to fuel my body, to make me as energized and strong as possible to withstand the demanding world of modeling.

I find grains, gluten, and dairy to be rough on my stomach, so I prefer to stick to a diet higher in protein and greens. This naturally led me on the path to a Paleo diet. It leaves my body feeling light.

I now feel so much stronger. My relationship with food is no longer one based on fear but is one of excitement, possibility, and fun!

NATIONALITY: Australian

LIVES IN: Los Angeles, CA, USA

CERTIFICATIONS: Institute for Integrative Nutrition Health Coach, Certified Intuitive Healer

FAVORITE WAYS TO MOVE: Pilates, spin class, nature hikes, yoga

KITCHEN MUST-HAVES: Spiralizer, cinnamon, turmeric, paprika, cumin, cayenne pepper

SEEN IN/KNOWN FOR: Aerie, American Eagle, Asos, Celine, Chloe, Lucky Brand, Free People blog, *Elle, Vogue, Marie Claire*

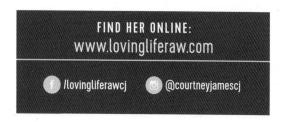

FIND HER ONLINE:
www.lovingliferaw.com

 /lovingliferawcj   @courtneyjamescj

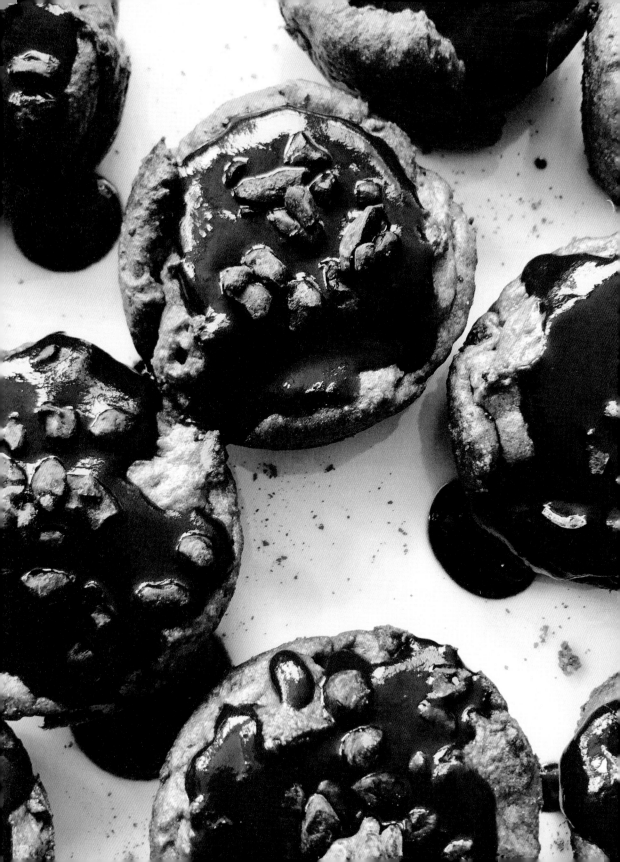

ENDLESS ENERGY MATCHA MUFFINS

I love matcha, or powdered green tea, as a coffee replacement. It gives me an even, sustained energy with no ugly crash afterward. These muffins are completely Paleo and use matcha powder for a delicious boost that also delivers a powerful dose of antioxidants. With this recipe, eating yummy baked goods doesn't have to be a guilty pleasure!

INGREDIENTS (10 Muffins):

MUFFINS

3 organic pasture-raised eggs

1 cup unsweetened coconut milk

½ cup extra-virgin coconut oil, melted

2 medium bananas (fairly ripe)

3 tablespoons granulated monkfruit sweetener (such as Lakanto)

1 teaspoon pure vanilla extract

1 tablespoon matcha powder

1¼ cups coconut or almond flour

2 teaspoons baking powder

Pinch of sea salt

Coconut oil cooking spray

GLAZE AND TOPPING

⅓ cup extra-virgin coconut oil

3 tablespoons pure maple syrup

2 tablespoons raw cacao powder

2–3 tablespoons cacao nibs (for topping)

DIRECTIONS:

MUFFINS

1. Preheat the oven to 350°F.
2. Combine the eggs, coconut milk, melted coconut oil, bananas, monkfruit sweetener, vanilla, and matcha powder in a blender and process until all the ingredients are incorporated
3. Whisk the flour, baking powder, and salt in a small bowl. Add to the liquid mixture in the blender and blend until well combined. The mixture should be quite runny and smooth.
4. Lightly grease 10 cups of a standard muffin tin with cooking spray, then divide the mixture evenly until nearly full.
5. Bake for 20 to 25 minutes, then transfer to a wire rack to cool.

GLAZE AND TOPPING

1. Heat the coconut oil in a saucepan over low heat just until melted. Mix in the maple syrup and raw cacao powder until smooth.
2. When the muffins have cooled, pour the glaze over and top with the cacao nibs.

CRUNCHY SUPERFOOD PALEO GRANOLA

I love adding crunch and a bit of sweetness to my chia seed pudding in the mornings, and this granola is ideal for that! I sprinkle it on top to give my breakfast extra nutrition for a more energized day. It is also an amazing snack to take while traveling or on the go!

INGREDIENTS (6 Servings):

5 tablespoons extra-virgin coconut oil, divided

⅓ cup raw honey

1 tablespoon ground cinnamon

1 tablespoon fresh lemon juice

3 cups gluten-free rolled oats

½ cup raw almonds

⅓ cup macadamia nuts

⅓ cup goji berries

½ cup unsweetened coconut flakes

1 tablespoon cacao powder

1 tablespoon maca powder

DIRECTIONS:

1. Preheat the oven to 325°F.
2. In a saucepan, combine 4 tablespoons of the coconut oil, the honey, cinnamon, and lemon juice, and bring to a boil over medium-high heat.
3. Remove from the heat and place in a large bowl. Add the oats, almonds, and macadamias and stir thoroughly to combine.
4. Line a rimmed baking sheet with foil, then grease the foil with the remaining 1 tablespoon coconut oil. Spread the granola on the sheet and bake for 35 minutes, stirring periodically.
5. Remove the granola from the oven and place in a large bowl. Add the goji berries, coconut flakes, cacao powder, and maca powder and mix well. Store in an airtight container until ready to use.

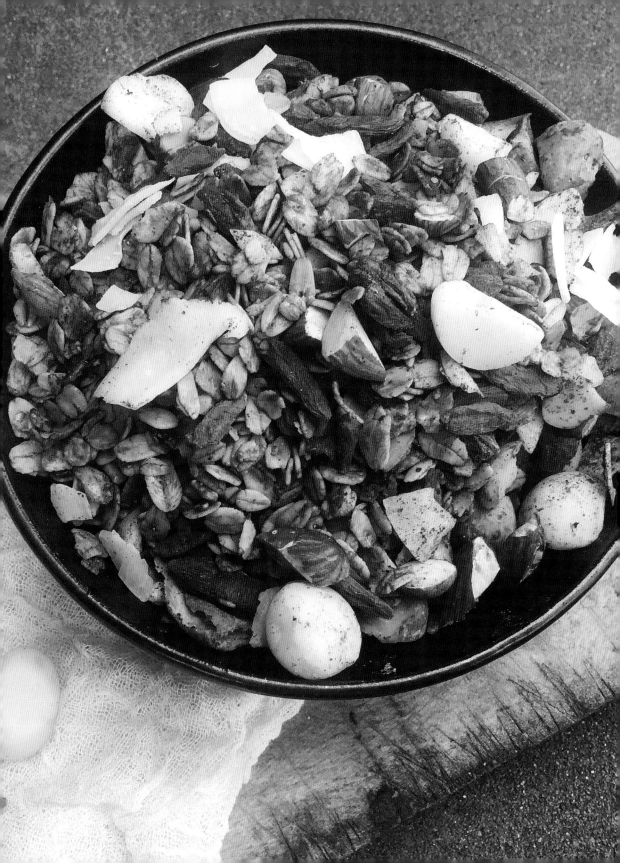

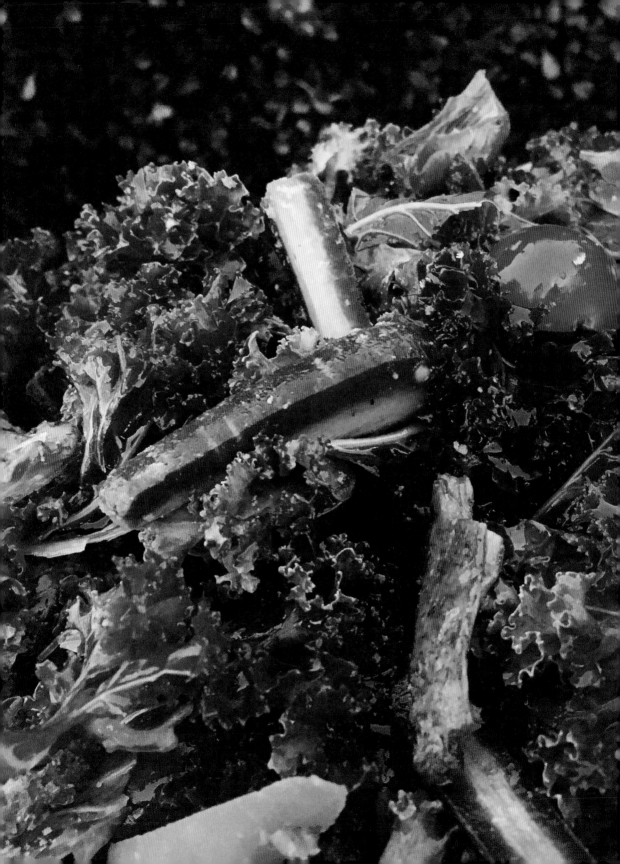

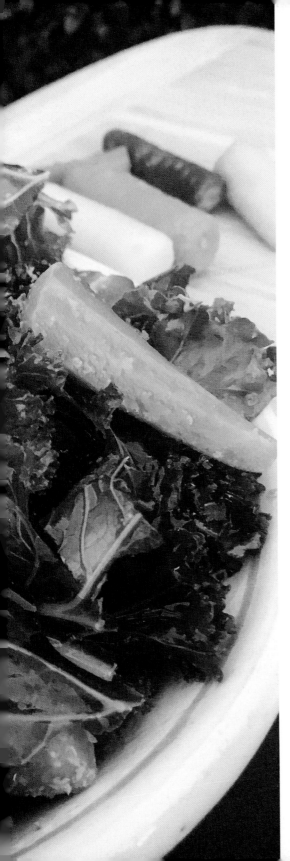

COLORFUL KALE SALAD

Kale is a nutritionally dense green with a satisfying bite. This salad is delicious and can easily accompany a meat or fish entrée, too. Including multiple colors will make any dish vary in nutrients and look prettier, making it more appealing and interesting to eat!

INGREDIENTS (3 Servings):

DRESSING

½ cup lemon juice
2 tablespoons extra-virgin olive oil
1 teaspoon apple cider vinegar
Salt and freshly ground black pepper, to taste

SALAD

1 bunch organic curly kale, stemmed and torn into bite-size
    pieces
1 cup sliced carrots
1 cup halved cherry tomatoes
¼ cup dried chili mango

DIRECTIONS:

DRESSING

1. Combine the lemon juice, olive oil, and apple cider vinegar in a large bowl, and season to taste with salt and pepper.

SALAD

1. Add the kale leaves to the dressing and massage to soften them and make them more easily digestible.
2. Mix the carrots, cherry tomatoes, and chili mango with the dressed kale leaves and toss to coat thoroughly with the dressing. Serve immediately and enjoy!

VEGAN RICE PAPER ROLLS

Rice paper rolls are a great appetizer for parties! Full of color, antioxidants, and vitamins, they're as deliciously refreshing as they are pretty.

INGREDIENTS (8 Servings):

1 bunch mint leaves

1 beet, scrubbed and grated or thinly sliced

1 mango, peeled, cored, and thinly sliced

1 avocado, peeled, pitted, and sliced

½ red bell pepper, thinly sliced

½ yellow bell pepper, thinly sliced

1 teaspoon extra-virgin coconut oil

8 slices tempeh

8 round rice paper wrappers

Dipping sauce of choice, for serving

DIRECTIONS:

1. Boil 3 cups of water and set aside to cool slightly.
2. In a large bowl, combine the mint, beet, mango, avocado, and bell peppers, and toss to combine.
3. Heat the coconut oil in a skillet over medium heat. Pan-fry the tempeh for 3 minutes on each side, or until golden brown.
4. Pour some of the hot water into a large shallow dish and submerge a rice paper wrapper to soften for 10 to 20 seconds.
5. Once soft, transfer the rice paper to a clean, slightly damp cutting board and gently smooth into a circle.
6. Add one-eighth of the vegetable filling and a slice of tempeh, then fold the bottom of the wrapper over the filling. Gently roll over again and fold in the sides to seal, then roll again until completely sealed. Place on a serving plate and cover with a damp towel to keep fresh.
7. Repeat the process with the remaining wrappers and filling. Serve with your favorite dipping sauce.

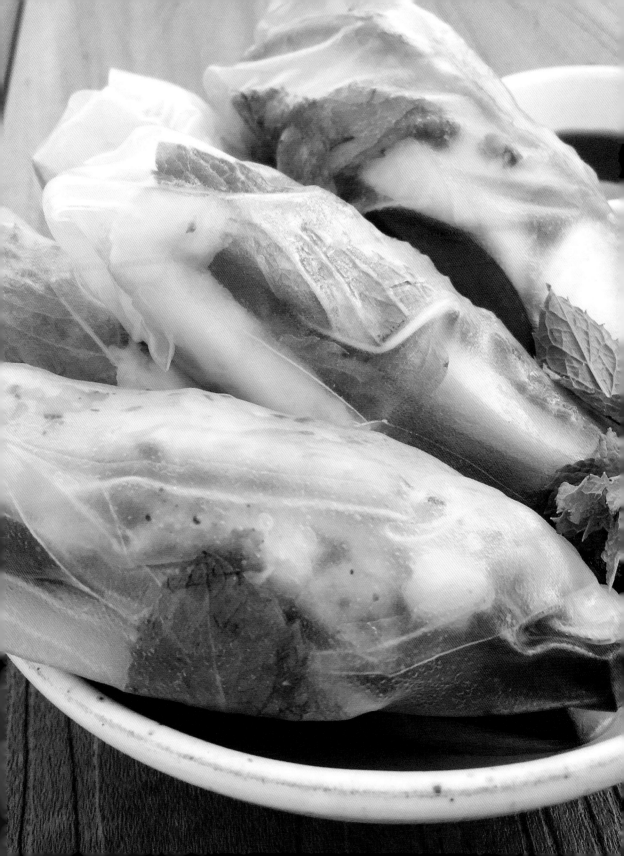

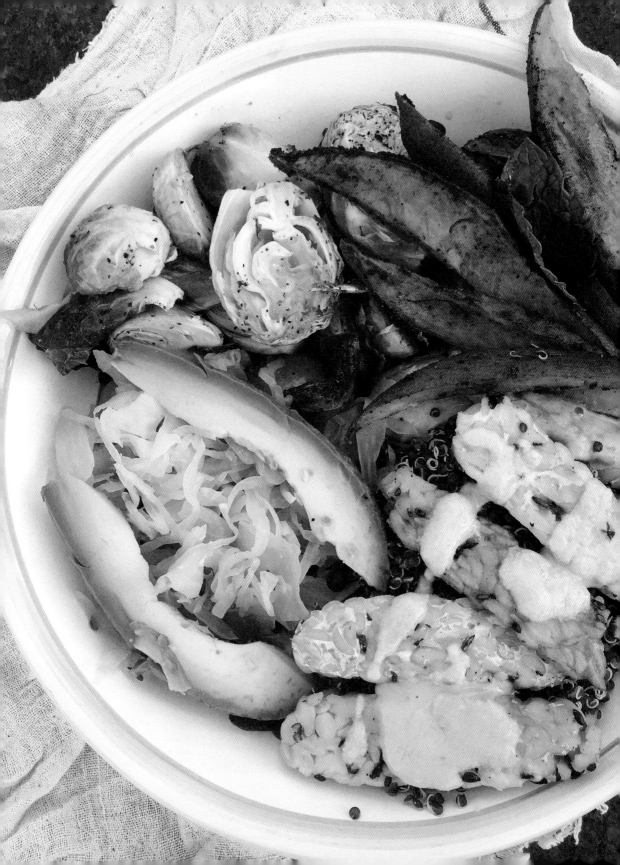

NOURISHING TEMPEH BOWL

This dish includes all my favorite flavors combined in one bowl! Roasted sweet potato chips, quinoa, greens, and coconut oil—fried tempeh are topped with tahini, homemade sauerkraut, and creamy avocado. It's a nourishing dish that never makes me feel bloated or too full, but warms the heart and body!

INGREDIENTS (1 Serving):

2 cups vegetable stock or water

1 cup tricolored or red quinoa, well rinsed

1 medium sweet potato, peeled and sliced into thin chips

2 tablespoons extra-virgin coconut oil, divided

¼ teaspoon sweet paprika

¼ teaspoon cayenne, divided

Pinch of sea salt

5 thin slices tempeh

2 cups dark leafy greens of your choice

1 teaspoon garlic salt

½ teaspoon ground turmeric

1 tablespoon tahini, for serving

½ Hass avocado, diced, for serving

¼ cup sauerkraut (page 90), for serving

DIRECTIONS:

1. Preheat the oven to 400°F. Line a baking sheet with foil.

2. In a saucepan, bring the stock to a boil. Stir in the quinoa and cook over high heat until the grains are soft and fluffy, 15 to 20 minutes. Transfer to a bowl and set aside.

3. In a bowl, toss the sweet potato chips with 1 tablespoon of the coconut oil, along with the paprika, half of the cayenne, and salt. Spread the chips on the prepared baking sheet and roast for 20 minutes, or until soft and golden.

4. Heat the remaining 1 tablespoon coconut oil in a skillet over medium heat and slightly brown the tempeh on both sides. Remove from the pan and set aside.

5. In the same skillet, lightly sauté the greens, seasoning with the garlic salt, turmeric, and remaining cayenne.

6. To serve, place the tempeh and greens over the quinoa and top with the sweet potato chips, tahini, avocado, and sauerkraut. Serve immediately and enjoy!

"A healthy body is crucial to also having a healthy mind, and I truly believe in balance and feeding ourselves in a way where we do not feel deprived. I'm passionate about living an authentic, conscious, and connected life and helping others feel more at peace, empowered, and healthy!"

AUTHENTIC RAW SAUERKRAUT

My mum is German, so she always had sauerkraut around, and this recipe has become a staple I use to add flavor, cultured probiotics, and vitamin C goodness to many meals and keep my gut on track. I love to use it in my Nourishing Tempeh Bowl (page 89) for that extra kick of fermented nourishment!

INGREDIENTS (12 Servings):

1 tablespoon sea salt

3 cups filtered water or celery juice

5 small or 3–4 large, dense cabbages, outer leaves separated and kept whole, inner leaves shredded in a food processor

12 medium-large carrots, peeled and grated

1 head Chinese bok choy, chopped

1 large red onion, chopped

Garlic cloves, peeled, to taste

DIRECTIONS:

1. Dissolve the salt in the water or celery juice and set aside.
2. Add the cabbage, carrots, bok choy, and onion to a large bowl and pound with a blunt tool to release their juices.
3. Stir the vegetables well, then add as many cloves of garlic as you like. Divide the mixture between clean glass jars, leaving 2 to 2½ inches of space at the top. Push the mixture down as far as possible to remove air bubbles, then top with a cabbage leaf, tucking it down over the top.
4. Pour the brine over the vegetables in each jar until they are fully submerged. If desired, use a weight, such as a small zip-top bag filled with brine, to hold the vegetables down during fermentation. Cover loosely with a two-piece canning lid.
5. Store the jars at room temperature for 28 days. Every 2 days, uncover and use a clean spoon to push the ingredients below the brine, allowing gas to escape from the jar and ensuring that the vegetables are fully submerged (if they are not, mix up a little more water and salt and add to the jar to prevent mold from forming).
6. Refrigerate after 28 days and enjoy!

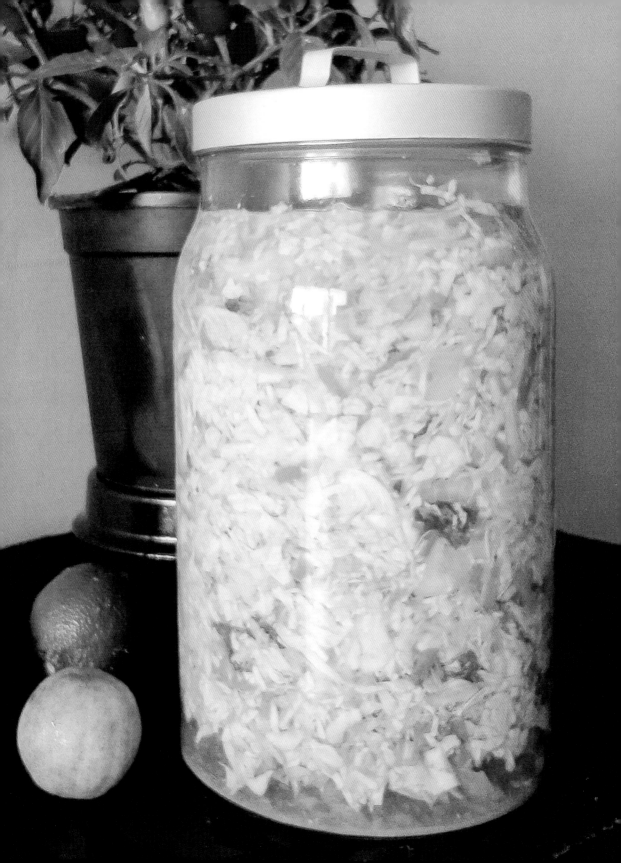

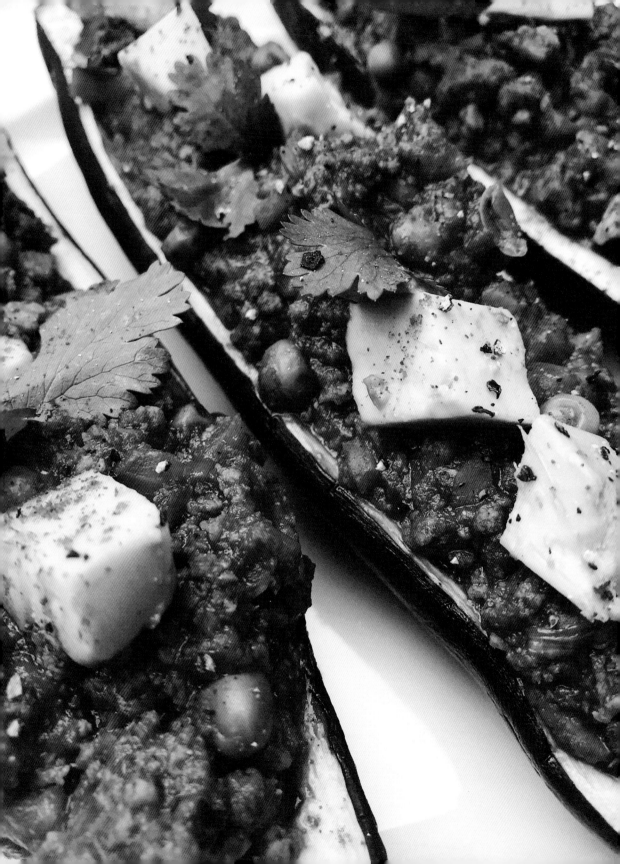

PALEO STUFFED ZUCCHINI BOATS

These zesty, delicious little boats are completely Paleo! Cook them on a grill or roast them in the oven—they're as versatile as they are nutritious.

INGREDIENTS (4 Servings):

4 large zucchini, halved lengthwise

1 tablespoon extra-virgin coconut oil

1 garlic clove, crushed

1 white onion, chopped

2 large carrots, chopped

1 cup frozen or fresh peas

1 pound ground beef

1 (15-ounce) can tomato sauce

1 (6-ounce) can tomato paste

½ teaspoon red pepper flakes

½ teaspoon cayenne

4 large fresh basil leaves, chopped

Sea salt, to taste

½ avocado, diced, for serving

½ cup chopped fresh cilantro, for serving

DIRECTIONS:

1. Preheat the oven to 375°F. Line a baking sheet with foil or parchment paper.

2. Using a spoon, scoop out the center of each zucchini half, being careful to not make the inside too thin. Place the zucchini halves on the prepared baking sheet and roast for 10 minutes.

3. In a large sauté pan, heat the coconut oil and garlic over medium-high heat. Add the onion, carrots, and peas and sauté until the veggies the are soft, 4 to 5 minutes.

4. Add the beef to the pan and cook until entirely golden brown, about 10 minutes. Stir in the tomato sauce, tomato paste, red pepper flakes, cayenne, and basil. Mix well to combine and season with salt.

5. Simmer for an additional 5 to 7 minutes, until the mixture thickens. Taste and adjust the spices if necessary.

6. Remove the zucchini from the oven and spoon the beef mixture into each boat. Top with avocado and cilantro. Serve immediately.

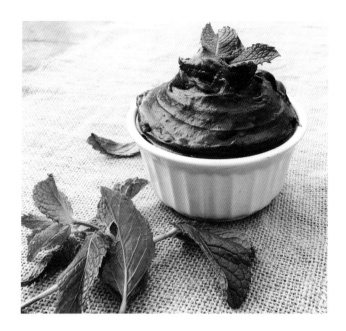

CHOCOLATE MOUSSE

I am secretly obsessed with both avocado and chocolate! This recipe is super easy to whip together and gives me a healthy chocolate fix after any meal.

INGREDIENTS (5 Servings):

2 large Hass avocados, peeled and pitted
5 tablespoons raw honey
⅓ cup raw cacao powder
1 teaspoon ground cinnamon
Pinch of sea salt
Fresh mint leaves, for garnish

DIRECTIONS:

1. Place the avocados, honey, cacao powder, cinnamon, and salt in a powerful blender and blend together. You can also use a whisk to whip the ingredients together in a bowl, but a blender gives the smoothest, most mousse-like texture.
2. Scrape into a bowl, garnish with mint, and serve immediately.

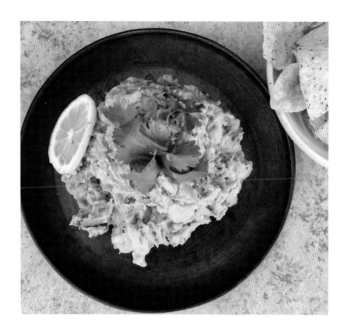

QUICK GUACAMOLE

This guacamole is so easy to prepare and packed with flavor and nutrition. Avocados provide the healthy fats that fuel our brain and give us long-lasting endurance, so enjoy them without guilt! Serve with vegetable slices and corn chips for dipping.

INGREDIENTS (6 Servings):

3 large Hass avocados, halved and pitted

Juice of 1 lemon

1 medium ripe Roma or heirloom tomato, finely chopped

¼ red onion, finely chopped

¼ cup finely chopped fresh cilantro, plus more for serving

1 garlic clove, crushed

Sea salt and freshly ground black pepper, to taste

DIRECTIONS:

1. Scoop the avocados from their skins and mash with a fork in a bowl.

2. Add the lemon juice, tomato, onion, cilantro, and garlic and gently mix until thoroughly combined. Season with salt and pepper.

3. Garnish with additional cilantro and serve immediately.

PALEO CHOCOLATE CHIP BANANA CAKE

Banana bread is a quintessential Australian sweet breakfast choice. We usually love eating it with walnuts, but this recipe is nut-free, as I personally love my banana bread smooth without the crunch. This bread is incredibly moist and works just as well as a no-guilt dessert!

INGREDIENTS (10 Servings):

¼ cup extra-virgin coconut oil, melted, plus more for the pan

3 bananas, plus more for serving

3 organic pasture-raised eggs

½ cup dark chocolate chips

¼ cup raw honey or 1 teaspoon stevia powder

¼ cup coconut flour

1 tablespoon pure vanilla extract

½ teaspoon baking soda

¼ teaspoon sea salt

Ground cinnamon, for garnish

DIRECTIONS:

1. Preheat the oven to 350°F. Grease a 9-inch bread pan with coconut oil.
2. In a large bowl, mash the bananas with a fork. Add the eggs, chocolate chips, coconut oil, honey or stevia powder, coconut flour, vanilla, baking soda, and sea salt and mix until the batter is smooth and silky.
3. Pour into the prepared pan and bake for 25 to 30 minutes, or until the bread is firm and beginning to develop a slight crust around the edges.
4. Remove from the oven and let cool, then serve with sliced bananas and a sprinkle of cinnamon.

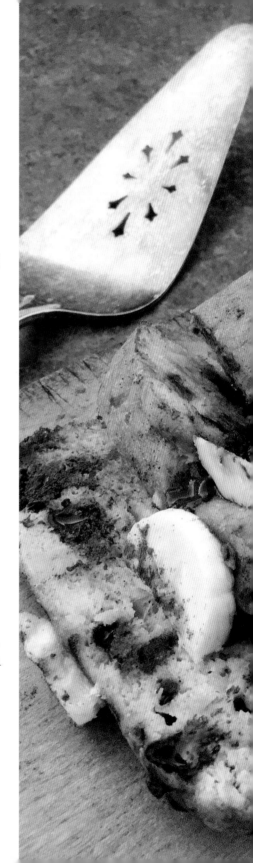

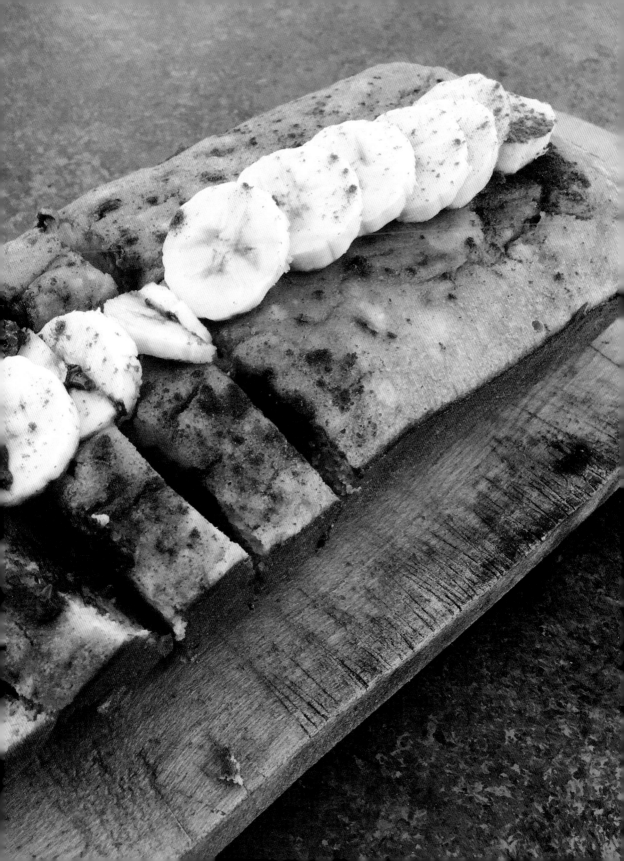

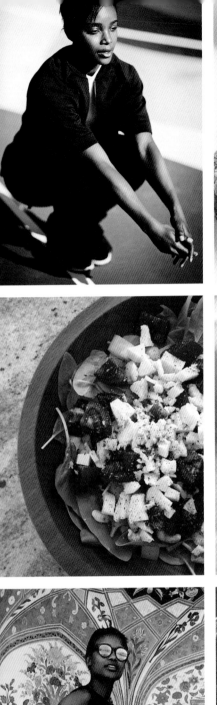
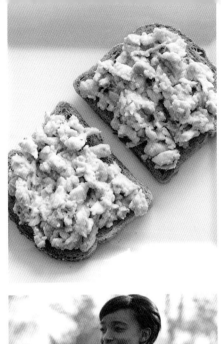
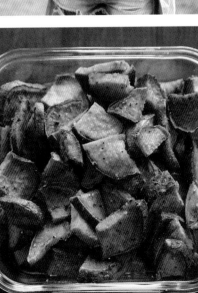
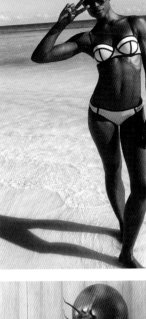
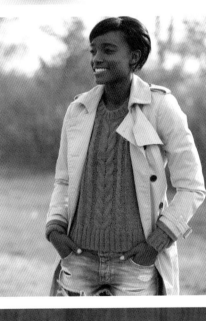
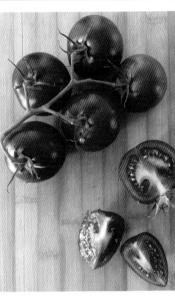
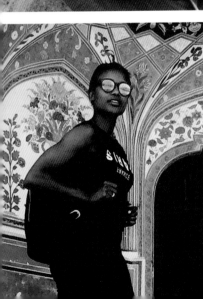
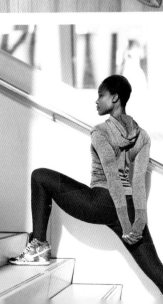

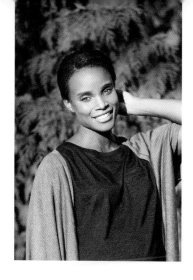

Simply Delicious

LAUREN WILLIAMS

There was a time when I was super focused on leaning out and lowering my body fat, and I think counting calories was very helpful for me then. It was more about gaining awareness of my eating habits. But since that brief period of counting calories, I've found other ways to improve my awareness and know exactly what I'm putting into my body, like preparing and cooking my own meals.

Failure is life's best teacher. I think I've spent most of my life trying not to make mistakes, afraid of doing the "wrong thing." I'm finally realizing there often isn't a "wrong," just many different paths and choices along the way. And even when you do make mistakes, those are the times you learn and grow the most—and they definitely make for the best life stories!

NATIONALITY: American/Bajan

LIVES IN: New York, NY, USA

CERTIFICATIONS: National Association of Sports Medicine

FAVORITE WAYS TO MOVE: Strength training, dance, high-intensity interval training (HIIT)

KITCHEN MUST-HAVES: Coconut oil, pink sea salt, cumin, garlic, cilantro, red pepper flakes

SEEN IN/KNOWN FOR: Nike, Athleta, Garnier, L'Oréal, Target, Kohls, *Glamour*, *Women's Health*, *Self*, *Shape*, *O Magazine*

FIND HER ONLINE:
www.chiselclub.com

🐦 @lajoy 224
f /lajoy224
📷 @lajoy224

🐦 @chiselclub_byla
f /chiselclub_bylauren
📷 @chiselclub_byla

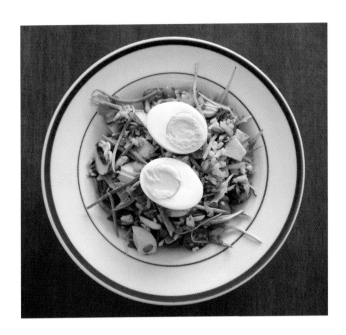

BREAKFAST SALAD

Salad for breakfast? Yes, you read that correctly! When my first meal is green-focused, I feel light and energized right up to lunchtime.

INGREDIENTS (4–6 Servings):

3 cups arugula
2 cups halved cherry tomatoes
2 cups shredded carrots
2 cups chopped mushrooms
1 cup cooked wild rice
½ cup sunflower seeds
½ cup sliced almonds
Extra-virgin olive oil, for drizzling
Balsamic vinegar, for drizzling
Sea salt, to taste
1–2 hard-boiled eggs per serving, halved

DIRECTIONS:

1. In a large salad bowl, combine the arugula, tomatoes, carrots, mushrooms, wild rice, sunflower seeds, and almonds.
2. Plate individual servings of the salad, and drizzle each with olive oil and balsamic vinegar, then season with salt to taste.
3. Top with sliced egg halves and serve.

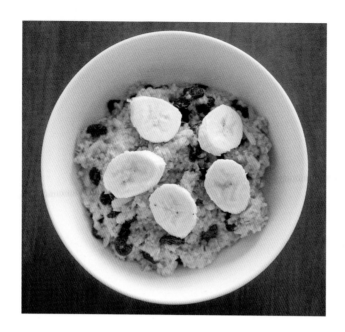

OVERNIGHT OATS

Save yourself some time in the morning by prepping breakfast the night before. I especially love it on days when my first workout of the day is going to be very intense or I'm hitting multiple workouts before lunch.

INGREDIENTS (2–4 Servings):

1 cup rolled oats

1 cup almond milk

⅛ teaspoon ground cinnamon

½ cup raisins

⅛ cup whole almonds

1–2 bananas, sliced

1 tablespoon raw honey (or to taste)

Pinch of salt

DIRECTIONS:

1. Mix together the rolled oats, almond milk, and cinnamon, then cover and refrigerate overnight.
2. The next morning, add the raisins, almonds, sliced banana, honey (if using), and salt. Mix together and enjoy.

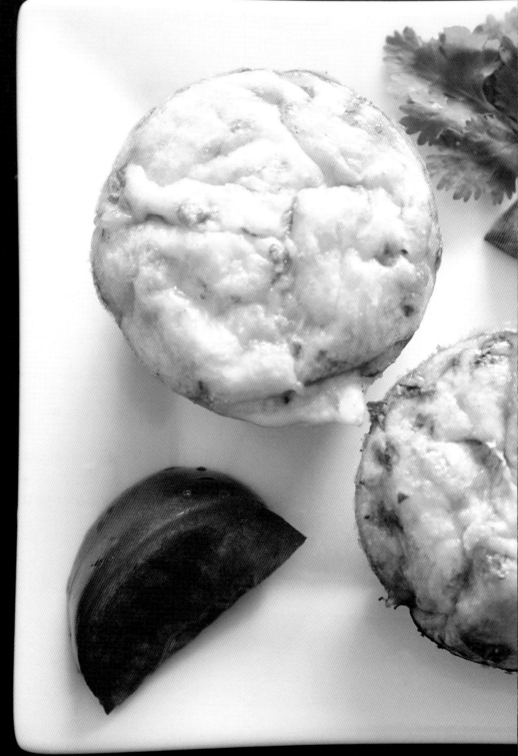

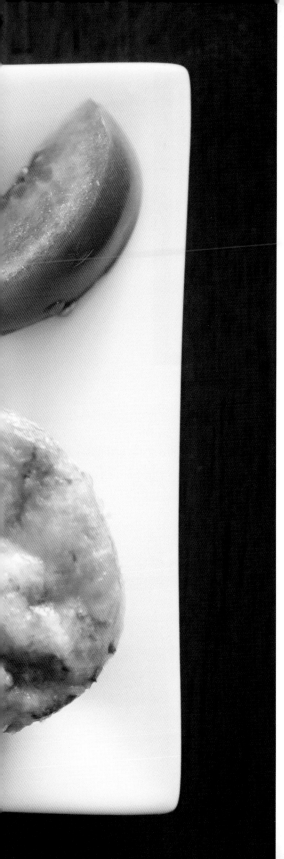

CILANTRO BREAKFAST EGG MUFFINS

I have many fond memories from childhood of my mother making her classic egg casserole dish on special mornings. So I was really excited to perfect this recipe with her! The cilantro adds a unique twist, and we took out the bread base layer to make it healthier. But the cheese still gives it a hearty, rich taste that is sure to wake you up. Baking it in muffin tins allows you to take it with you anywhere, anytime.

INGREDIENTS (6 Muffins):

Butter, for the muffin tin
3 organic pasture-raised eggs, beaten
¾ cup grated sharp cheddar cheese
½ cup 2 percent milk
½ teaspoon powdered mustard
1 tablespoon finely chopped fresh cilantro leaves
6 ounces chicken apple sausage, chopped

DIRECTIONS:

1. Preheat the oven to 350°F. Grease 6 cups of a standard muffin tin lightly with butter.
2. In a large bowl, combine the eggs, cheddar cheese, milk, powdered mustard, and cilantro, and beat with a whisk. Set aside.
3. Lightly brown the sausage over low heat. Sprinkle into the bottom of the prepared muffin tin cups, then pour the egg mixture over the top.
4. Bake for 24 to 28 minutes, until the eggs are firm. Enjoy!

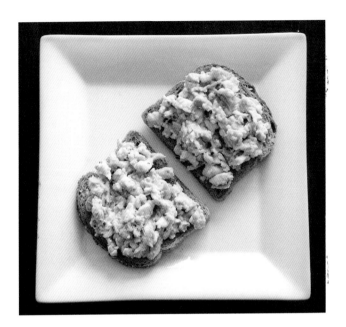

AVOCADO TOAST

Who doesn't love the health benefits of avocado, such as potassium, healthy fatty acids, and fiber? There is research to show that healthy fats like avocado can help the body absorb vitamins from other foods, so consider pairing this delicious toast with a salad for extra nutrition.

INGREDIENTS (1 Serving):

1 avocado, halved and pitted
Juice of ½ lemon
½ tablespoon extra-virgin olive oil
1 teaspoon garlic salt, or to taste
1 teaspoon red pepper flakes, or to taste
2 slices multigrain bread

DIRECTIONS:

1. In a small bowl, mash the avocado by hand and squeeze the lemon over it. Add the olive oil and mix well. Add the garlic salt and red pepper flakes to taste.
2. Toast the bread to your preference and spread the avocado mixture thickly over it. Serve immediately.

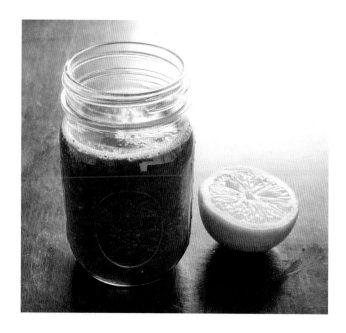

CHERRYBERRY SMOOTHIE

Smoothies are my breakfast go-to in the summertime, and my post-workout staple after strenuous sessions. This recipe combines fruits that are both rich in antioxidants and great for replenishing energy. Add protein powder to aid in muscle recovery.

INGREDIENTS (2 Servings):

2 cups spinach

1 cup frozen cherries

1 cup coconut milk

1 cup frozen blueberries

½ medium banana

1 scoop protein powder (optional)

Fresh lemon juice, to taste

DIRECTIONS:

1. Place the spinach, cherries, coconut milk, blueberries, banana, and protein powder (if using) in a blender and blend to the desired consistency. Add lemon juice to taste, and then blend once more to combine. Serve immediately.

SPICY COLLARDS AND CABBAGE SALAD

Want to shake up your salad routine? This is the recipe for you.
Instead of spinach or arugula, why not try something out of
the ordinary, like collard greens and cabbage? I love the taste
and the texture of this salad! The sweet and spicy dressing
complements the raw vegetables beautifully. To make it a more
filling meal, add a protein like a piece of baked fish or quinoa.

INGREDIENTS (2–4 Servings):

SALAD
4 cups thinly sliced collard greens
1 cup thinly sliced red cabbage
1 yellow or red bell pepper, cored, seeded, and thinly sliced
Optional proteins: baked fish, quinoa

DRESSING
½ cup extra-virgin olive oil
2½ tablespoons raw honey
1½ tablespoons sriracha sauce
1½ teaspoons garlic powder
½ teaspoon lemon juice, freshly squeezed
½ teaspoon ground ginger

DIRECTIONS:

1. In a large salad bowl, combine the collard greens, cabbage, and
    bell pepper.
2. In a separate, smaller bowl, whisk the dressing ingredients together
    until well combined and emulsified.
3. Add the dressing to the salad and mix thoroughly. Top with your
    protein of choice (if using) and serve immediately.

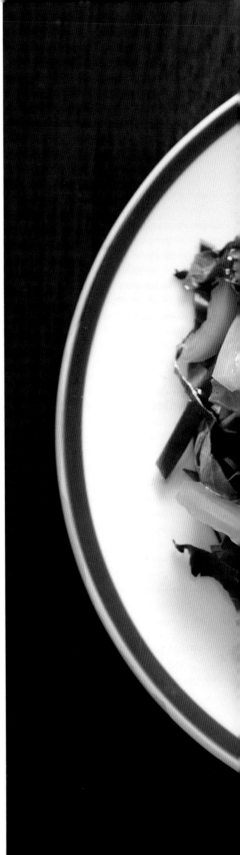

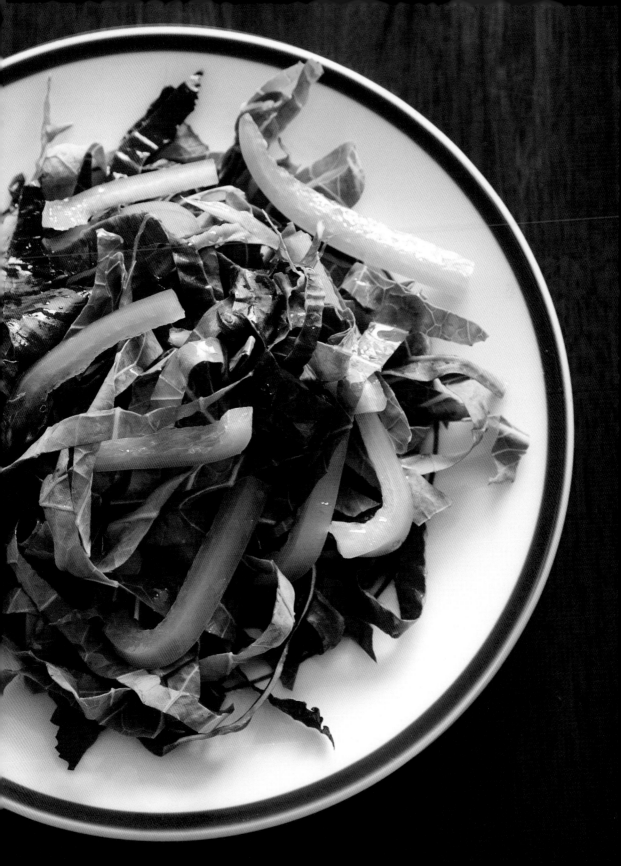

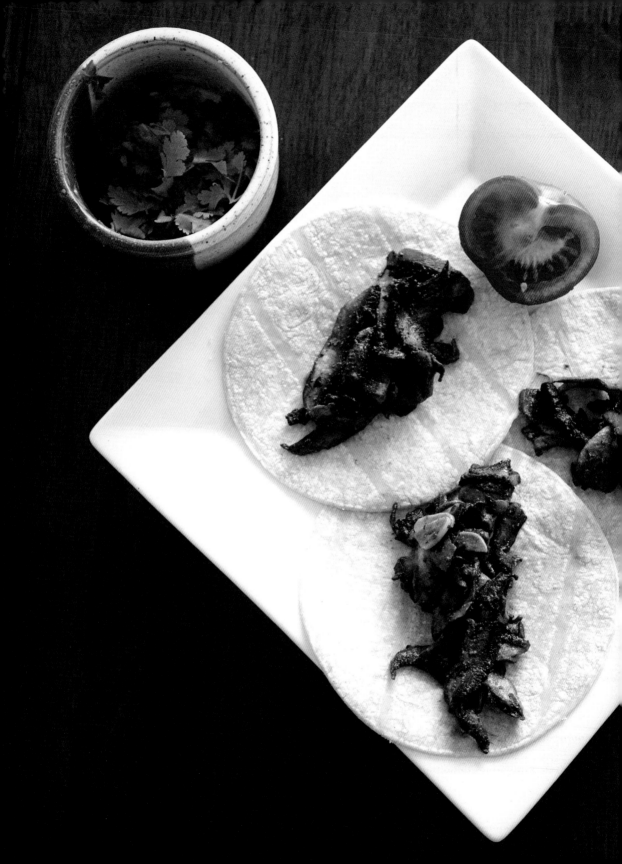

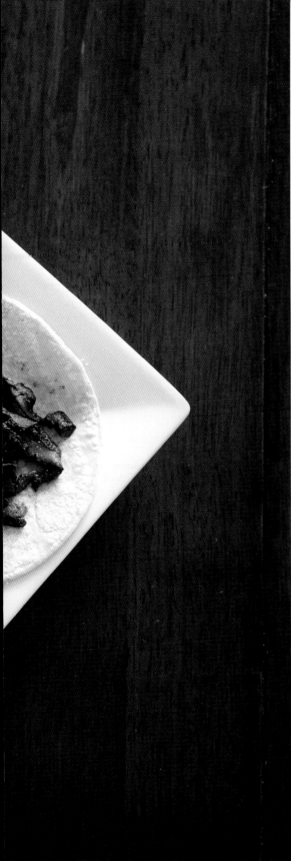

WHOLESOME MUSHROOM TACOS

Tacos are great anytime and the perfect dish to serve to a group. Building each little package by hand is a team effort that brings everybody to the kitchen! The mushroom filling in these tacos has a great texture that will satisfy meat lovers and vegetarians alike.

INGREDIENTS (4 Servings):

2 tablespoons extra-virgin olive oil
3 garlic cloves, crushed
1 cup sliced portobello mushrooms
1 cup sliced shiitake mushrooms
1 cup sliced cremini mushrooms
3 teaspoons ground cumin
Sea salt and ground black pepper, to taste
8 corn tortillas, warmed
½ cup chopped fresh cilantro leaves

DIRECTIONS:

1. In a large sauté pan, heat the olive oil over medium-high heat and add the garlic, stirring to coat. When the garlic starts to brown, add the mushrooms and reduce the heat to medium.
2. Cook for 3 to 6 minutes, or until the mushrooms are soft and glossy.
3. Add the cumin and combine thoroughly, coating the mushroom mixture well, then season with salt and pepper.
4. Serve immediately with warmed tortillas and top with cilantro.

GINGER CHILI SAUTÉ

I find I can greatly simplify my weekly cooking process by prepping ingredients at the beginning of the week and storing them for later. For this recipe, I chop the vegetables and tofu on Sunday night and keep each serving in a plastic bag in the fridge. When I get home from a long day of teaching, training, or shooting, all I have to do is reach in the refrigerator for a bag and throw it into a pan on the stove. Dinner is served in less than 20 minutes!

INGREDIENTS (4–6 Servings):

4 tablespoons sesame oil

3 garlic cloves, thinly sliced

3 tablespoons grated fresh ginger

1 teaspoon red pepper flakes, plus more for serving

½ teaspoon lemon juice

1 cup thinly sliced carrots

3 cups chopped broccoli

1 yellow bell pepper, cored, seeded, and chopped

1 cup chopped shiitake mushrooms

1 (14-ounce) package firm tofu, rinsed and cut into 1-inch cubes (optional)

Sea salt, to taste

DIRECTIONS:

1. In a sauté pan over medium heat, heat the sesame oil. Add the garlic, fresh ginger, and red pepper flakes and cook until the garlic just begins to brown. Add the lemon juice and stir together.

2. Add the carrots, broccoli, bell pepper, and mushrooms to the pan and sauté for 5 to 10 minutes, until soft.

3. Stir the tofu (if using) into the vegetable mixture and season with salt and more red pepper flakes to taste. Continue to cook until heated through and serve immediately.

"Food is so many things to me. It's nourishment, it's comfort, it's celebration, it's relief, it's joy. Of course, there are times when food brings up feelings of anxiety. But mostly, food is one of the joys of life. It gives me fuel to do the things I love and a chance to commune with friends and family. It is fun, and it is satisfying."

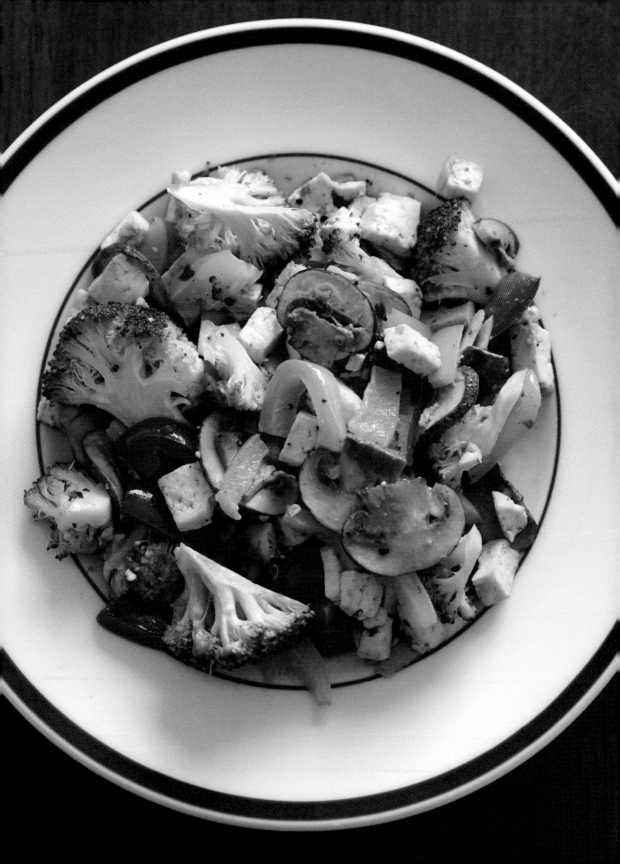

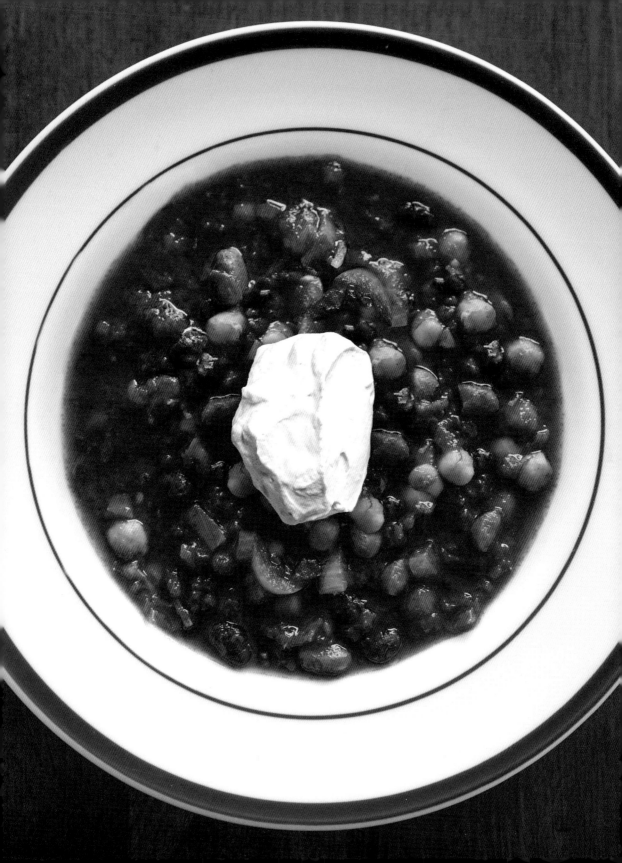

THREE-BEAN CHIPOTLE CHILI

Chili is a winter staple in my kitchen. It's healthy, hearty, and delicious—perfect for taking the cold weather chill out of my body! This recipe adds a smoky, slightly spicy twist to traditional chili that pulls all the flavors together. I make it in a slow cooker for convenience, but you can also slow cook it on the stove. Just be sure to stir it often to keep it from sticking on the bottom.

INGREDIENTS (4–6 Servings):

3 tablespoons extra-virgin olive oil
1 cup diced onion
5 garlic cloves, crushed
1 (15-ounce) can chickpeas, rinsed and drained
1 (15-ounce) can black beans, rinsed and drained
1 (15-ounce) can white beans, rinsed and drained
2 (7.5-ounce) cans tomato sauce
1 (7-ounce) can chipotles in adobo sauce
1½ cups water
1 teaspoon sea salt
1 teaspoon freshly ground black pepper
1 teaspoon red pepper flakes
Plain Greek yogurt, for topping (optional)

DIRECTIONS:

1. In a slow cooker, heat the olive oil on high. Add the onion and garlic and cook for approximately 2 minutes.
2. Add the beans and tomato sauce, cover, and let cook for 30 minutes.
3. Remove the chipotles from their sauce and chop them. Add the chopped chipotles, adobo sauce, water, salt, pepper, and red pepper flakes. Cover and let cook for 3½ hours.
4. Plate the chili and top it with a generous dollop of yogurt for added creaminess, if desired.

CURRIED FISH STEW

I'm a big fan of curries and spicy foods from different cultures around the world. This curried fish stew is one of my favorites; after much experimentation with the seasonings, I've created a recipe that is colorful and savory, pleasing to both the eye and the palate.

INGREDIENTS (6–8 Servings):

6 garlic cloves, crushed, divided

4 tablespoons freshly squeezed lemon juice

4 tablespoons extra-virgin olive oil, divided

1 pound cod fillets, cubed

1 cup chopped onion

½ yellow bell pepper, diced

½ red bell pepper, diced

2 cups chopped tomatoes

4 tablespoons curry powder

2 teaspoons sea salt

1 teaspoon freshly ground black pepper

1 (14-ounce) can coconut milk

½ cup chopped fresh cilantro leaves, for serving

½ cup chopped scallions, for serving

DIRECTIONS:

1. In a large bowl, mix 3 garlic cloves with the lemon juice and 1 tablespoon of the olive oil. Add the cod and stir thoroughly, then set aside to marinate.

2. In a large skillet with a lid, heat the remaining 3 tablespoons olive oil over medium-high heat and sauté the onion, bell peppers, and remaining 3 garlic cloves until soft.

3. Add the tomatoes, curry powder, salt, and pepper and stir thoroughly. Reduce the heat to low, cover, and simmer for 15 minutes.

4. Remove the cod from the marinade and add it and the coconut milk to the pot; stir to combine. Cover and simmer for 20 to 30 minutes, or until the fish is completely cooked. Remove from the heat and let stand for 5 minutes.

5. Garnish with cilantro and scallions and serve immediately.

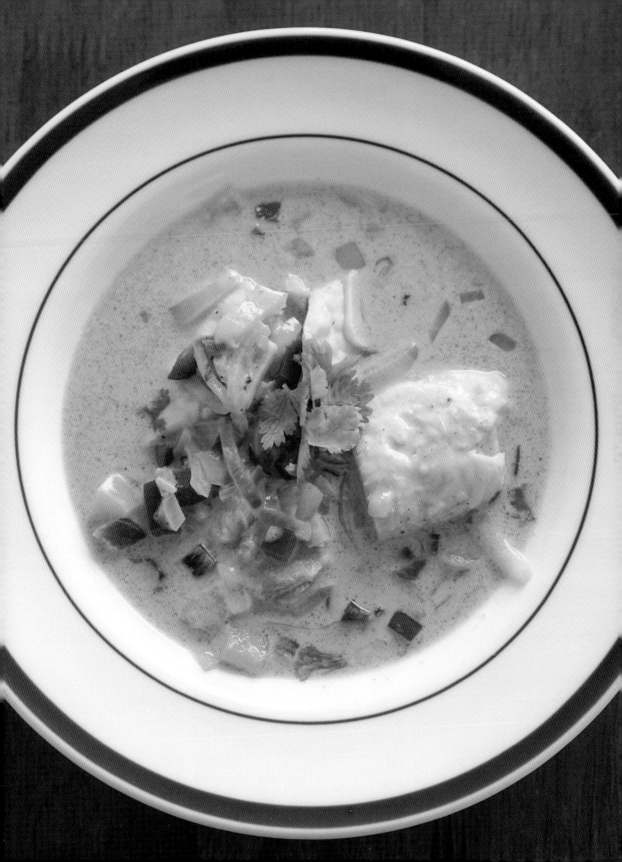

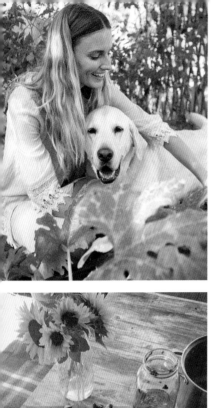
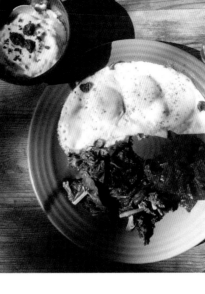
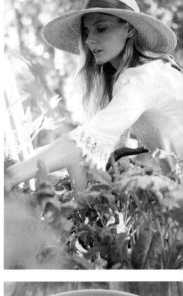
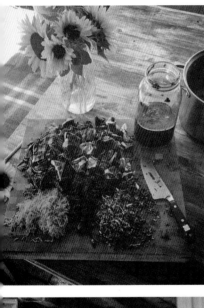
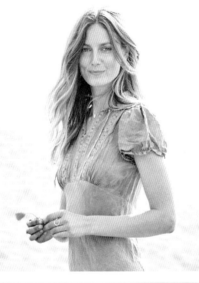
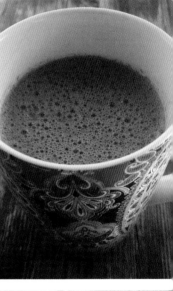
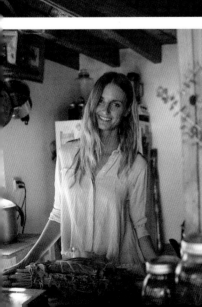
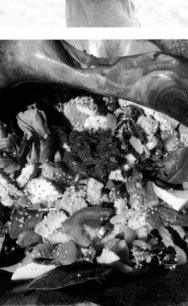
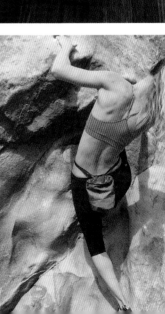

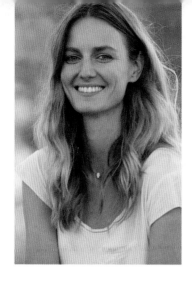

Happy Belly

COLLEEN BAXTER

Through most of my fashion modeling career, I was indoctrinated to fear fullness or curves, and even strength and muscle tone. It never felt like my body was just right. My agents told me I had to stop backpacking and rock-climbing, and eventually that hit a nerve. I chose "health and happiness" as my mantra, and decided that as long as I was eating healthy and exercising and felt good, then I would accept and love my body as it was.

My cooking philosophy is grounded in the rich healing powers of nature. My body- and mind-nourishing recipes are pre- or probiotic rich and nutrient dense, and support overall energy and well-being. As we balance the gut and hormones with healing foods and flavors, we can better tune in to our body and internal wisdom, and live with more peace, joy, and purpose.

NATIONALITY: American

LIVES IN: Topanga, CA, USA

CERTIFICATIONS: Functional Medicine Certified Health Coach (FMCHC), National Board Certified Health and Wellness Coach (NBC-HWC), Certified Lifestyle Educator (LE)

FAVORITE WAYS TO MOVE: Hiking with my dogs, yoga, rock-climbing with friends

KITCHEN MUST-HAVES: Vitamix, turmeric, cinnamon, cayenne, garlic, sea salt, olive oil

SEEN IN/KNOWN FOR: *Vogue, Elle, Harper's Bazaar, Numéro, The Devil Wears Prada*, TJ Maxx. Runway: Armani, Oscar de la Renta, Monique Lhuillier

FIND HER ONLINE:
www.vesselandsoul.com

@vesselandsoul   @vesselandsoul

/VesselAndSoul

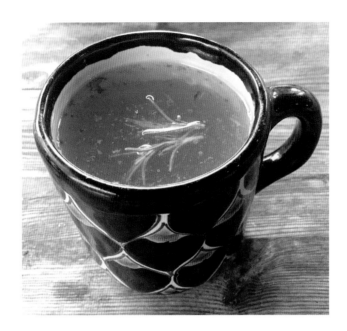

BONE BROTH

Bone broth is one of the most nourishing foods in existence. Packed with essential minerals like calcium, magnesium, and phosphorus, as well as vital nutrients like glucosamine, chondroitin, gelatin, and essential fatty acids, it's a golden elixir of youth.

INGREDIENTS (10–12 cups):

3 pounds bones (preferably grass-fed/pasture-raised bison or beef marrow bones or pasture-raised organic chicken bones)

Filtered water, to cover (about 4 quarts)

2 tablespoons sea salt

1 tablespoon apple cider vinegar

Optional: chopped vegetables and herbs, such as onions, carrots, celery, parsley, rosemary, thyme, seaweed, and nettle

DIRECTIONS:

1. Place all the ingredients in a large pot on the stove. Bring to a simmer, then let cook at your stove's lowest setting for 12 to 72 hours. The longer you cook the bones, the more minerals and nutrients will be pulled from them.

2. Discard the bones, strain out any solids, carefully pour the broth into mason jars with vacuum-seal lids, and store in the refrigerator. The broth will keep for about 5 days in the refrigerator or can be frozen for several months.

3. To serve, warm gently and use as a base for soups and stews, or just drink as a healthy tonic first thing in the morning.

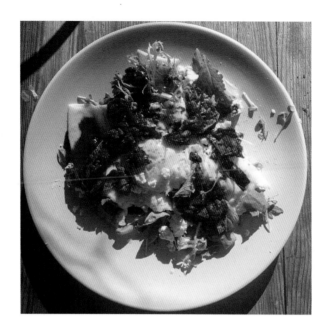

EGGSELLENT MORNING

Pasture-raised eggs, cooked over-easy to provide vital choline and cholesterol from the raw yolk, are a complete protein with good fats for healthy hormone balance, brain function, and lasting fuel. Paired with cultured vegetables and sautéed kale, this is a beautifully balanced breakfast that is rich in the building blocks for a healthy, happy, and more hormonally balanced woman.

INGREDIENTS (1 Serving):

1 tablespoon grass-fed butter or ghee
2 organic pasture-raised eggs
1 tablespoon extra-virgin coconut oil
1 handful of kale leaves, stems removed, chopped
Cultured Vegetables (page 120), for serving
Sea salt, to taste

DIRECTIONS:

1. Melt the butter in a cast-iron pan over low heat. Crack the eggs into the pan and cover with a lid, allowing the whites to cook and the yolks to remain raw.
2. In another pan, or after the eggs have been removed from the pan and plated, melt the coconut oil over medium-low heat. Add the kale, pour in a tiny bit of water, cover with a lid, and cook for about 1 minute.
3. Plate the eggs with the sautéed kale and a side of cultured vegetables, then sprinkle gently with a little salt and enjoy!

CULTURED VEGETABLES

Cultured or fermented vegetables are easy for the body to digest, improve the digestion of other foods, and are packed with pre- and probiotics to cleanse and nourish gut flora. Cheap to make, this staple is a zesty and beneficial complement to eggs, meat, and veggie dishes.

INGREDIENTS (8 Servings):

1 head organic cabbage
Optional vegetables and flavorings: carrot, beet,
 horseradish root, ginger, garlic, green beans, dill
1–3 tablespoons sea salt
Filtered water

ADDITIONAL SUPPLIES:

1-quart mason jar with vacuum-seal lid

DIRECTIONS:

1. Wash your hands and the vegetables, and sanitize the mason jar, a cutting board, knives, and a large bowl with soap and hot water to ensure a clean environment for healthy fermentation.
2. Remove the first two outer leaves of the cabbage and discard. Gently remove the next two leaves and set aside for later. Then shred, chop, or food-process the cabbage along with any of the optional vegetables (if using), and place in the large bowl. Pour in the sea salt. With your hands, mix and massage the vegetables, again and again, until the cabbage is turning translucent and you have a good amount of vegetable liquid in the bowl.
3. Pack the mixture into the jar, pressing down on the vegetables to remove any air and leaving about 3 inches of space to the top of the jar. Pour in the liquid brine from the bowl to completely cover the vegetables plus ½ inch. If you need additional liquid to cover, you can add salt water.
4. Press a reserved cabbage leaf into the jar, tucking it and pushing down to ensure the vegetables are submerged. Use a chunk of cabbage or carrot, a glass fermentation weight, or a boiled river stone, and place on top to weigh down the mixture, so it remains fully submerged while fermenting.
5. Seal the jar with a two-piece canning lid and place in a cool, dark area.
6. Check in every 3 days. Remove the lid to allow air to escape, use a clean spoon to ensure that the vegetables are completely submerged, and taste to see if it has reached the desired fermentation. This can take anywhere from 3 to 7 weeks, depending on the temperature of your kitchen, the produce used, etc. It's ready when it's fizzy and tastes sour and crunchy to your liking.
7. When ready, store in the refrigerator, and eat as a condiment throughout the day for a happy gut. It will stay good in your refrigerator for up to 8 months, but you should enjoy consuming it well before then.

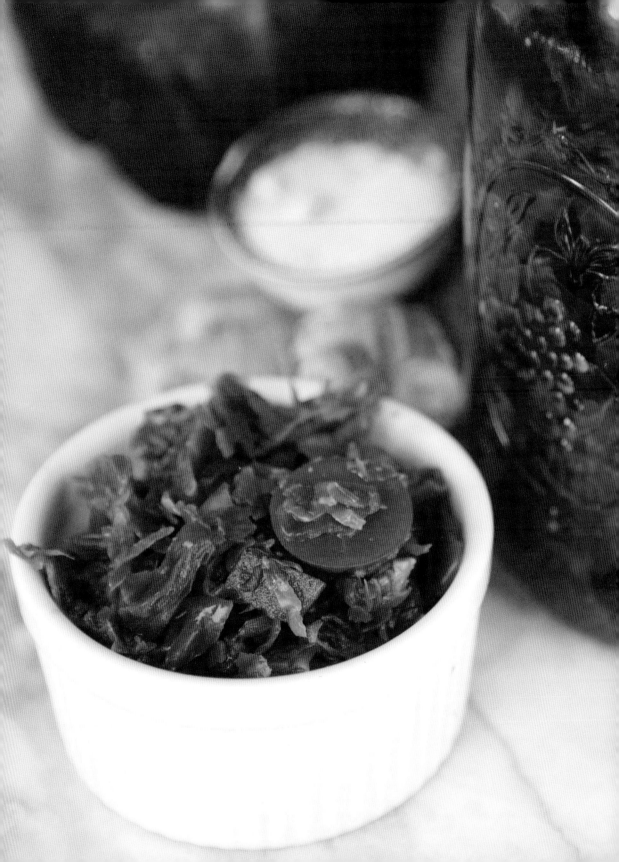

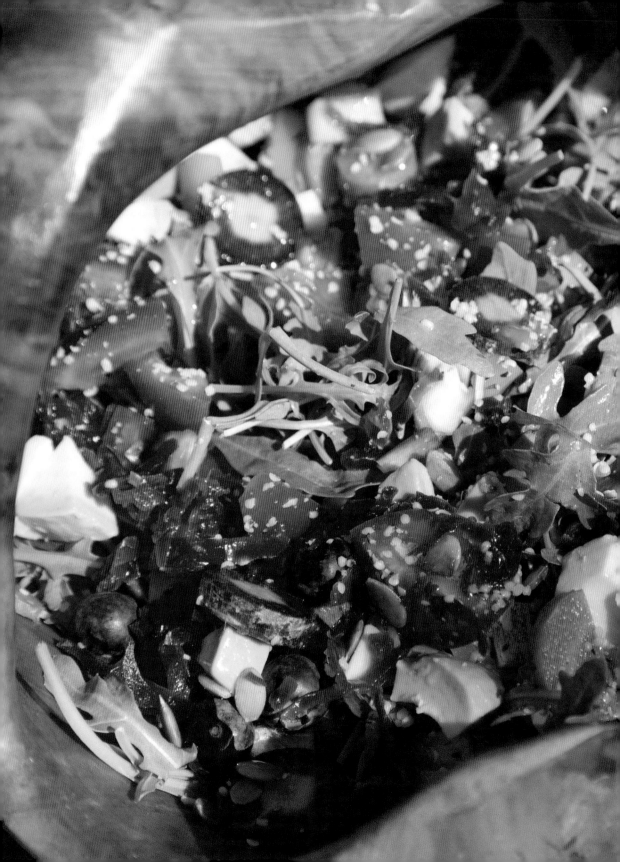

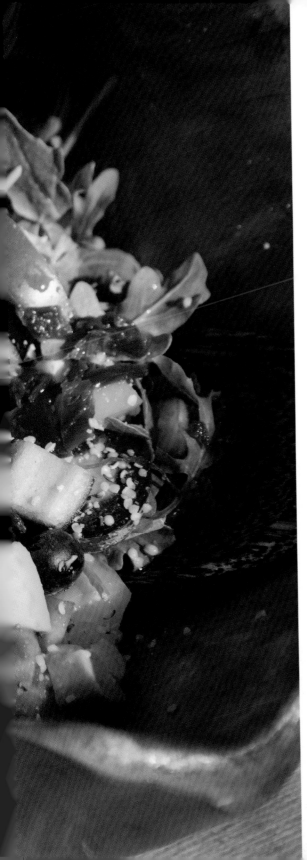

RAINBOW SALAD

The more variety and richness of natural colors in our diet, the greater the phytonutrient and antioxidant content; these help fight free radicals and other contributing factors to disease. This salad is full of color, flavor, and richness and is also both detoxifying and healing. Try to make all your salads and meals rich in color and variety. Eating healthy never has to be boring! Eat as is, or top with an over-easy egg, wild-caught fish, or other high-quality protein.

INGREDIENTS (4 Servings):

4 cups wild arugula (or other salad greens)

1 avocado, peeled, pitted, and diced

1 heirloom tomato, diced

½ orange bell pepper, diced

¼ red onion, diced

⅓ cup blueberries

Juice of 1 lemon

2 tablespoons extra-virgin olive oil

¼ cup raw pecans, chopped

2 tablespoons hemp seeds

¼ cup Cultured Vegetables (page 120)

DIRECTIONS:

1. Combine the arugula, avocado, tomato, bell pepper, onion, and blueberries in a large salad bowl.
2. Pour on the lemon juice and olive oil, then sprinkle with the pecans and hemp seeds.
3. Mix the salad, top with the cultured vegetables, and serve!

BISON STEW

Using the Bone Broth recipe on page 118, we can make this incredibly delicious and nutritious stew. It's particularly nourishing for the time around a woman's menses, but the men in your life will love it, too. With the richness of bioavailable iron, plus healthy fats and protein, this stew is blood-building, hormone-balancing, comforting, and nourishing to the vessel and soul.

INGREDIENTS (5 Servings):

12 cups Bone Broth (page 118)

1–2 sweet potatoes, peeled and chopped

1 onion, chopped

5 garlic cloves, crushed

2 handfuls spinach

1 carrot, chopped

1 sprig fresh rosemary, chopped

2 tablespoons organic grass-fed ghee (or extra-virgin coconut oil if avoiding dairy)

1 pound grass-fed ground bison meat

Cayenne, to taste

Sea salt, to taste

Optional garnishes: diced avocado, fresh parsley, fresh cilantro

DIRECTIONS:

1. In a large pot, combine the bone broth, sweet potatoes, onion, garlic, spinach, carrot, and rosemary. Bring to a low boil over medium-high heat. Reduce the heat and simmer for approximately 40 minutes.

2. In a cast-iron pan over medium-low heat, melt the ghee, add the bison, stir to mix thoroughly, and cover. Cook until the meat is evenly browned, stirring occasionally.

3. Add the bison to the broth and vegetable mixture and cook over low heat for another 15 minutes. Season to taste with cayenne and salt. Garnish as desired and enjoy!

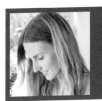 "I was so incredibly shy growing up. I've since found a stronger fire within and place myself in challenging situations to speak up, be free, and allow my quirky authentic self to shine whenever I feel it trying to hide or doubt its worthiness."

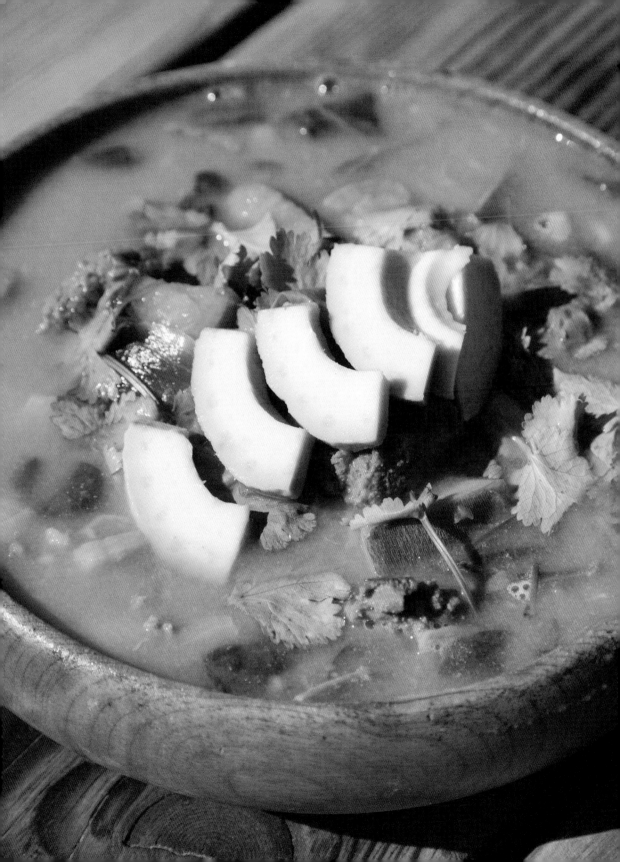

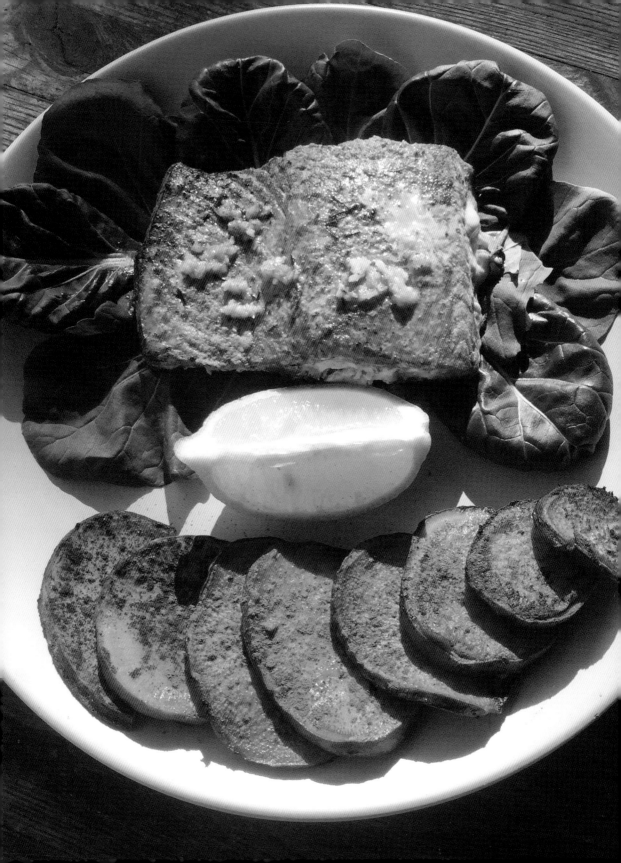

SPICED SALMON WITH SWEET POTATOES

This dish is full of healthy fats and vibrant spices to fuel your hormones, mind, and libido. The kale and sweet potatoes are great nutrient-rich fiber sources for healthy digestion and also balance blood sugar. Basically, this meal is so good, you won't know what to do with your sexy self.

INGREDIENTS (2 Servings):

Juice of ½ lemon

½ teaspoon paprika

¼ teaspoon sea salt, plus more as needed

¼ teaspoon ground black pepper

¼ teaspoon ground turmeric

¼ teaspoon cayenne

Pinch of saffron

2 wild salmon fillets, fresh or thawed

3 tablespoons extra-virgin coconut oil, divided

1 sweet potato, peeled and sliced

4 tablespoons filtered water

1 tablespoon ground cinnamon

3 garlic cloves, crushed

Lemon wedges, for garnish

DIRECTIONS:

1. In a dish large enough to hold both fillets in a single layer, whisk together the lemon juice, paprika, salt, pepper, turmeric, cayenne, and saffron. Place the salmon fillets flesh side down in the marinade, cover, and refrigerate for 15 minutes.

2. Melt 2 tablespoons of the coconut oil in a skillet over low heat. Line the pan with the sweet potato slices and add the water. Sprinkle with the cinnamon and 2 pinches of sea salt, cover, and cook over low heat until tender while you prepare the salmon.

3. Melt the remaining 1 tablespoon of the coconut oil in a second skillet over medium-low heat. Remove the salmon from the marinade, reserving the marinade, and place in the skillet, skin side down; pour the marinade over the top. Smear the crushed garlic on top of the salmon, cover with a lid, and cook over low heat for 5 to 10 minutes, or until firm.

4. Plate the fish and potatoes with a wedge of fresh lemon for squeezing and serve immediately.

FERTILE FEMME ICE CREAM

This ice cream is dangerous only because it's entirely guilt-free, and thus you may find yourself making variations of it and wanting to eat ice cream all day, every day. It's packed with delicious healthy fats that help balance your metabolism and hormones, stabilize blood sugar, increase libido, and make you feel like the decadent goddess you are.

INGREDIENTS (4 Servings):

1 tray coconut milk ice cubes (12 cubes, made from canned or fresh coconut milk)

2 egg yolks from organic pasture-raised eggs

¾ cup organic grass-fed plain kefir

½ cup full-fat coconut milk

¼ cup cacao powder

1 tablespoon xylitol

1 tablespoon grass-fed ghee or extra-virgin coconut oil

1 tablespoon grass-fed collagen powder

⅔ teaspoon peppermint extract

¼ teaspoon chocolate stevia

Pinch of sea salt

½ teaspoon pearl powder (optional)

Optional garnishes: fresh mint leaves, cacao nibs, goji berries, golden berries, chopped nuts

DIRECTIONS:

1. Combine the coconut milk cubes, egg yolks, kefir, and coconut milk in a high-powered blender, starting on low, and gradually increase the speed until thoroughly blended, using the blender tamper wand as needed.

2. Add the cacao powder, xylitol, ghee or coconut oil, collagen powder, peppermint extract, chocolate stevia, salt, and pearl powder (if using) and blend completely. If necessary, add a little water or coconut milk to thin the mixture.

3. If the ice cream is too soft, use an electric ice cream maker to increase firmness, or just enjoy as is.

4. Garnish as desired and serve immediately.

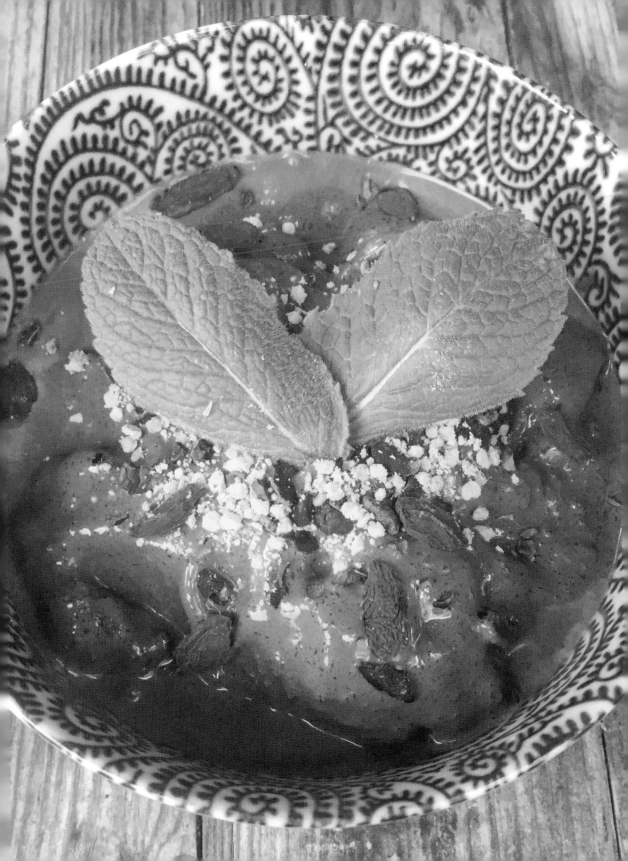

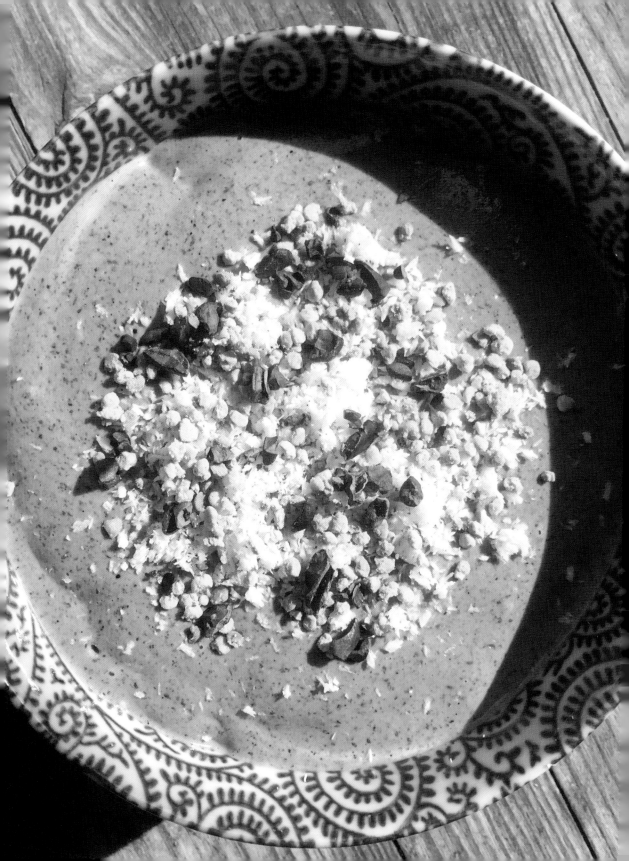

CHIA CACAO PUDDING

This warm pudding is delicious as a dessert or can be a meal on its own, because it's a no-guilt, nourishing delight. The chia base is wonderful for fiber and smooth movement through the gut. The healthy fats are great for gut and brain function, hormone balance, and satiety. Customize it by experimenting with different flavors if spiced chocolate isn't your favorite.

INGREDIENTS (2 Servings):

1 cup organic coconut milk

½ cup filtered water

¼ cup chia seeds

2 tablespoons cacao powder

1 tablespoon grass-fed whey or collagen protein powder

1 tablespoon extra-virgin coconut oil

1 tablespoon grass-fed ghee

½ teaspoon vanilla bean powder

½ teaspoon organic liquid stevia

1 teaspoon xylitol

½ teaspoon ground cinnamon

2 pinches of cayenne

½ teaspoon ginger juice

Optional toppings: bee pollen, nuts, seeds, fresh fruit

DIRECTIONS:

1. In a pot, gently warm the coconut milk and water over low heat. When it's warm to the touch, remove from the heat and add the chia seeds. Stir until thickened.

2. Add the chia mixture and the remaining ingredients to a blender. Start blending on low speed and increase gradually to high until smooth. Pour into bowls.

3. Add the toppings of choice and enjoy!

MOJITO COCONUT YOGURT

As you can tell, I am a huge fan of fermented raw foods, and fresh coconut yogurt is a deliciously creamy way of getting these beneficial probiotics into the gut for a healthy, vibrant body. Commercial yogurts are made from pasteurized dairy, often loaded with sugar and artificial flavorings. This coconut yogurt is raw, has no added sugar, is packed with probiotics, and serves as a treat that's both healthy and delicious.

INGREDIENTS (2 Servings):

Meat of 3 fresh coconuts

Juice of ½ lemon

1 teaspoon vanilla bean powder

1 heaping tablespoon finely chopped fresh mint leaves

1 tablespoon coconut kefir water (optional)

Fresh coconut water

2 probiotic capsules (ideally a broad-spectrum blend)

Optional toppings: chopped cacao nibs, chopped macadamia nuts, bee pollen

DIRECTIONS:

1. In a high-powered blender, combine the coconut meat, lemon juice, vanilla bean powder, mint, kefir water (if using), and enough coconut water to blend smoothly.

2. Open the probiotic capsules, pour the contents into the blender, and blend until dissolved.

3. Scoop the yogurt into a dish, add toppings of choice, and eat as a tasty dessert. Or, for a bigger health boost, scoop into mason jars (fill only halfway), twist on lids to seal, and let sit on the countertop to ferment for 3 to 6 hours. Chill and serve as a super probiotic-rich sour coconut yogurt.

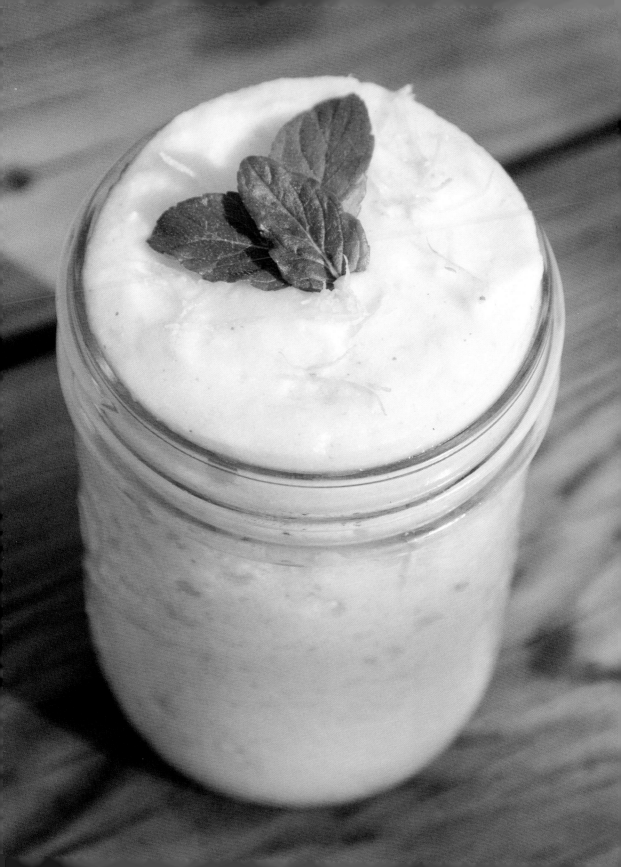

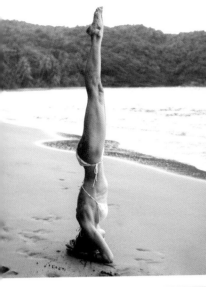
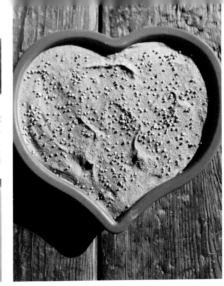
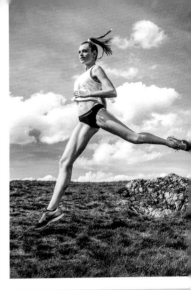
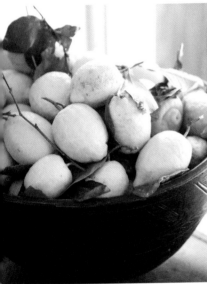
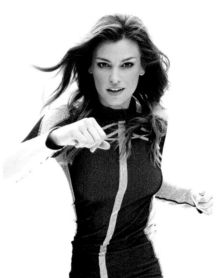
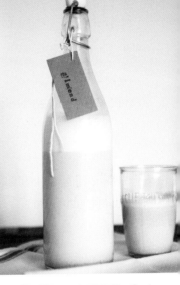
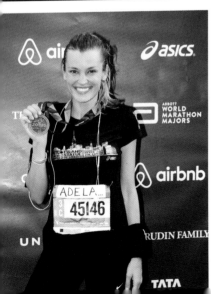
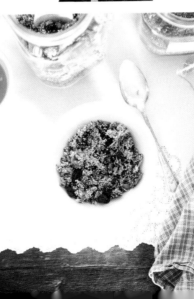
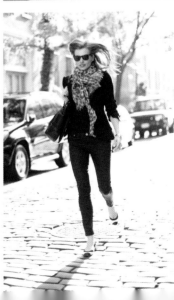

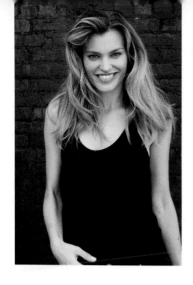

Fitness Fuel

ADELA CAPOVA

I was discovered on a Prague subway by a modeling agent and shortly after signed a contract. I was in high school one minute and all set to start medical school when I graduated; the next minute I was flying around Europe—to Athens, Istanbul, and Hamburg—before settling in Milan. It didn't take long for me to realize that juggling medical school with modeling was going to be impossible.

I was always a curvy girl. I'm only 5-foot-8 and, even at the age of sixteen, I was called fat to my face by agency staff more than once. Their advice was to only drink water and eat apples.

Then I found running. I started packing my sneakers whenever I traveled and squeezing in a run whenever I could. The benefits were obvious; I felt happier, more active, fitter, and more positive. I started looking at food as fuel and treating my body like an athlete, not a model.

NATIONALITY: Czech

LIVES IN: New York, NY, USA

CERTIFICATIONS: Institute for Integrative Nutrition, AADP Drugless Practitioner, NASM Fitness Trainer

FAVORITE WAYS TO MOVE: Running, dance cardio, Pilates, yoga, kickboxing

KITCHEN MUST-HAVE: Lemons

SEEN IN/KNOWN FOR: Wonderbra, L'Oréal, Gap, Avon, Nivea, Clairol, H&M, Vichy, Lovable, *Elle*, *Vogue*, *Harper's Bazaar*, *Cosmopolitan*, *GQ*

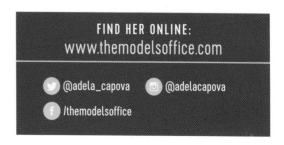

FIND HER ONLINE:
www.themodelsoffice.com

🐦 @adela_capova   📷 @adelacapova

f /themodelsoffice

BODYBUILDER'S BREAKFAST

This is my dad's everyday breakfast. When I first saw him eating it, I was very skeptical—but then I tried it! This meal has incredible nutritional value and uses sardines, a concentrated source of omega-3 fats that is also rich in vitamin B12 for a healthy heart, and vitamin D, the sun vitamin. Being a small fish and at the bottom of the aquatic food chain, sardines don't concentrate mercury and other toxins like other fish can. If you like savory breakfasts, this will be heaven for you. If not, be brave and try it anyway—you'll love it!

INGREDIENTS (2 Servings):

1 avocado, peeled, halved, and pitted
8 ounces boneless, skinless sardines packed in extra-virgin
    olive oil, drained
Juice of ½ lemon
1 tablespoon capers
2–3 tablespoons finely chopped fresh flat-leaf parsley
Pinch of sea salt
1 (15-ounce) can black beans, rinsed and drained

DIRECTIONS:

1. In a bowl, mash the avocado until smooth.
2. Add the sardines, lemon juice, capers, and parsley, and mix thoroughly.
3. Season with salt to taste and serve with black beans on the side.

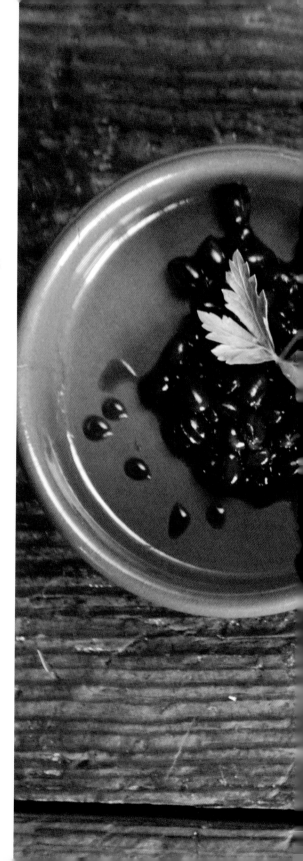

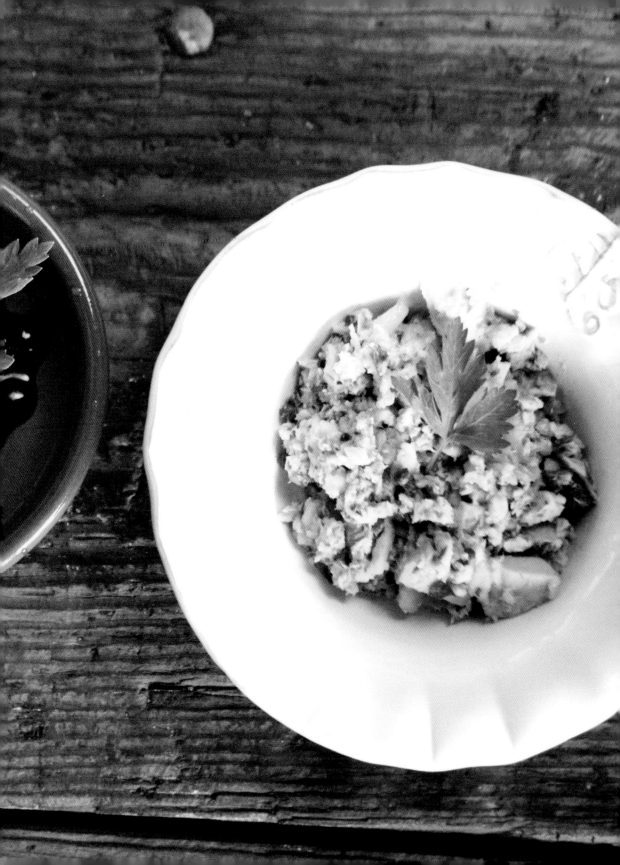

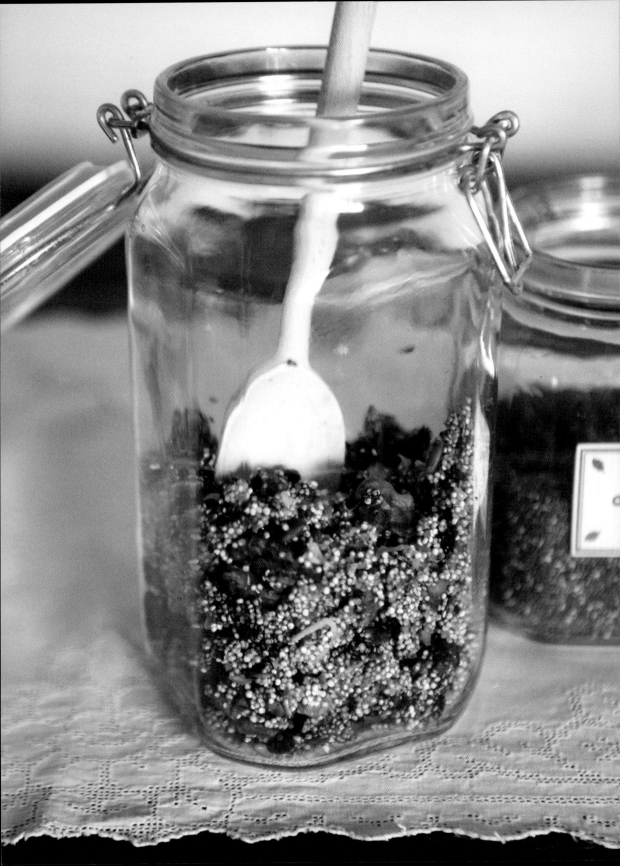

RUNNER'S GRANOLA

This healthy quinoa granola is truly yummy, and you can add any nuts, fruits, and seeds that you like. High in protein, it also has omega-3 fatty acids thanks to walnuts, flaxseeds, pumpkin, and chia seeds. Bake up a batch to keep on hand for breakfast or a snack—bonus: your house will smell amazing!

INGREDIENTS (7 Servings):

2 teaspoons extra-virgin coconut oil

1 handful walnut halves

¼ cup coconut flakes

2 tablespoons chia seeds

2 tablespoons flaxseeds

2 tablespoons pumpkin seeds

½ teaspoon ground cinnamon

½ teaspoon sea salt

1 cup quinoa, rinsed well

⅓ cup unsweetened applesauce

½ teaspoon raw honey

½ teaspoon pure vanilla extract

½ cup raisins (optional)

DIRECTIONS:

1. Preheat the oven to 350°F. Line a baking sheet with parchment paper.
2. Warm the coconut oil in a small pan and set aside.
3. Mix the walnuts, coconut flakes, chia seeds, flaxseeds, pumpkin seeds, cinnamon, and salt in a mixing bowl. Stir in the quinoa and set aside.
4. In another mixing bowl, mix the melted coconut oil, applesauce, honey, and vanilla.
5. Mix the wet and dry ingredients together, then spread the mixture evenly on the prepared baking sheet.
6. Bake for 20 to 25 minutes, stirring occasionally, until golden brown.
7. Add the raisins (if using), mix well, and refrigerate in an airtight container for up to 2 weeks.

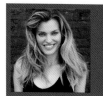

"I was born in the Czech Republic toward the end of communism. Something as simple as having a banana was a very special treat, so the idea of traveling around the world, experiencing new cultures and foods, was just beyond a dream. Getting paid for it was even more amazing!"

MORNING STRAWBERRY GOODNESS

This is my morning classic, especially in the summertime when I'm in the mood for something cold and refreshing. It's fast and easy to make, and will keep hunger at bay throughout the morning.

INGREDIENTS (2 Servings):

BASE

1 handful cashews, soaked in filtered water for at least 4 hours

1 handful Brazil nuts, soaked in filtered water for at least 4 hours

2 Medjool dates, pitted

2 tablespoons extra-virgin coconut oil, melted

Pinch of sea salt

PARFAIT

20 strawberries

1 handful cashews, soaked in filtered water for at least 4 hours

½ cup coconut milk (homemade, see below, or canned)

Juice of ½ lemon

1 tablespoon extra-virgin coconut oil, melted

HOMEMADE COCONUT MILK (OPTIONAL)

2 cups unsweetened shredded coconut

4 cups hot water (not boiling)

2 Medjool dates, pitted and soaked in filtered water until soft

½ teaspoon pure vanilla extract

DIRECTIONS:

BASE

1. Rinse the nuts thoroughly and drain them well. Blend all the base ingredients in a blender until almost smooth, with a few chunks left throughout.

PARFAIT

1. Wash the blender and blend all the parfait ingredients until smooth and creamy.

2. Divide the base mixture between two small bowls and flatten gently with a spoon.

3. Divide the parfait mixture in half and top each base evenly. There should be about 2 inches of parfait in each bowl.

4. Refrigerate for at least 1 hour before serving. Store overnight for a nutritious breakfast in the morning.

HOMEMADE COCONUT MILK

1. Blend the coconut and hot water in a blender until creamy (make two batches if it won't all fit).

2. Place cheesecloth or a nut milk bag over a large bowl and pour the mixture through. Pour the liquid in the bowl back into the blender (discarding the solids), add the dates and vanilla, and blend until creamy.

3. Store in an airtight container in the refrigerator for up to 5 days. Shake well before serving.

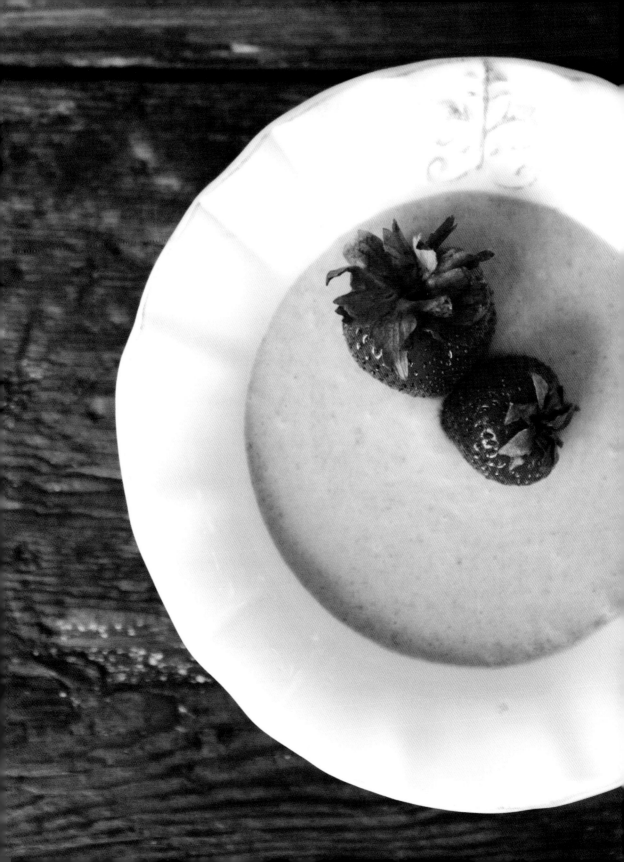

BROWN RICE SOUFFLÉ

Rice soufflé is a typical sweet Czech dish that I grew up eating. We serve it for lunch and sometimes dinner, too. In my country, it's usually cooked with white rice; I make it with brown rice and replace the sugar and a few other ingredients to make a healthier version. This delicious, nourishing entrée is always a big hit with kids!

INGREDIENTS (4 Servings):

1 cup brown rice, rinsed

4 cups coconut milk

4 organic pasture-raised eggs, separated and whisked thoroughly in two separate bowls

1–2 tablespoons pure maple syrup, to taste

1 teaspoon ground cinnamon

Pinch of sea salt

4 nectarines, pitted and chopped

Extra-virgin coconut oil, for the baking dish

DIRECTIONS:

1. Preheat the oven to 400°F.
2. In a large saucepan, cover the rice with the coconut milk and bring to a boil. Reduce the heat and simmer for 30 minutes, or until the rice is soft. Set aside and let cool.
3. In a large bowl, mix the cooled rice, egg whites, maple syrup, cinnamon, and salt. Gently fold in the nectarines.
4. Grease an 8 × 8-inch baking dish with coconut oil and add the rice mixture, topping with the beaten egg yolks.
5. Bake for 30 minutes, or until golden brown. Serve immediately and enjoy!

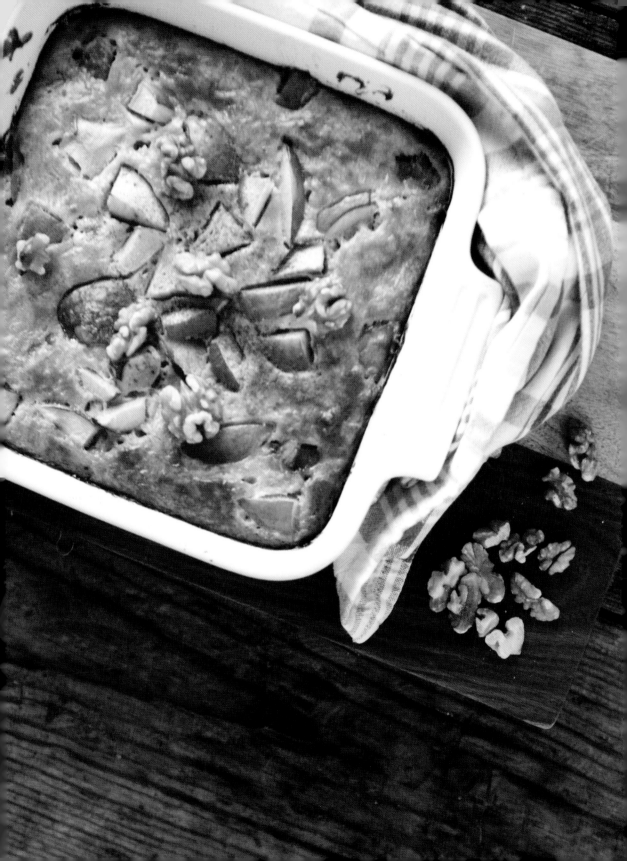

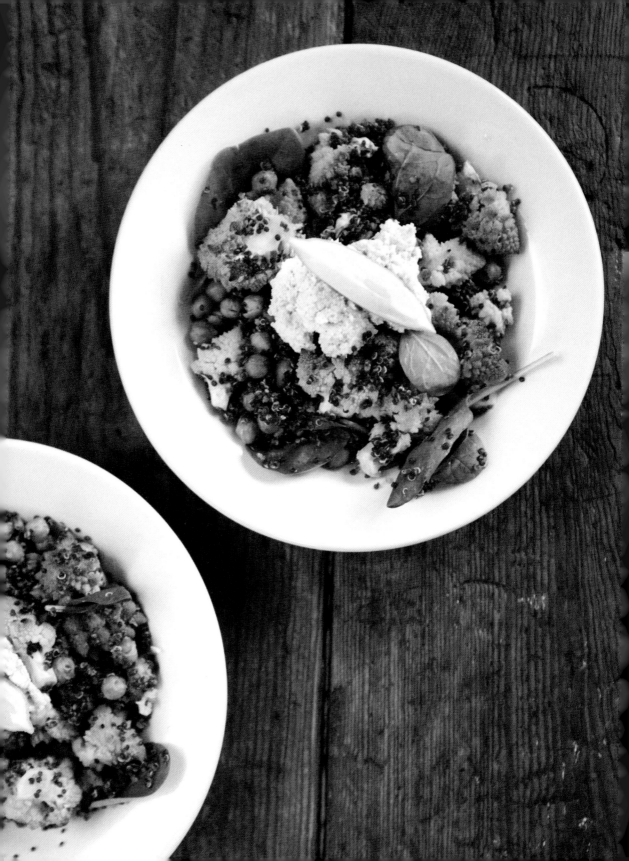

RUNNER'S QUINOA LUNCH

What I like most about this dish is the colors! A variety of color offers more nutrition, and this dish is filling but not overwhelming. I like to make it on a Sunday night and eat it during the week, or bring it on a plane. It's a perfect on-the-go lunch, packed with nourishment and energy.

INGREDIENTS (4 Servings):

QUINOA BOWL

1 head cauliflower or romanesco, chopped into medium-size florets

1 (15-ounce) can chickpeas, rinsed and drained

Extra-virgin olive oil

1 cup red quinoa, rinsed

1¾ cups vegetable stock

4 cups spinach

Sea salt and freshly ground black pepper, to taste

Lemon wedges, for serving

CASHEW RICOTTA

1½ cups raw cashews, soaked in filtered water for at least 4 hours and rinsed well

Juice of 1 lemon

1 garlic clove, crushed

1 tablespoon raw apple cider vinegar

Sea salt and freshly ground black pepper, to taste

DIRECTIONS:

QUINOA BOWL

1. Preheat the oven to 400°F and line a large baking sheet with parchment paper.
2. Spread the cauliflower and chickpeas evenly on the prepared sheet and sprinkle with enough olive oil to lightly coat.
3. Bake for 45 minutes, tossing every 15 minutes to cook evenly.
4. Meanwhile, place the quinoa in a medium pot and cover with the vegetable stock. Bring to a boil, reduce the heat to low, cover, and simmer for 12 to 15 minutes, or until the quinoa is fluffy.
5. In a large bowl, combine the chickpea and cauliflower mixture, cooked quinoa, spinach, salt, pepper, and a drizzle of olive oil.

CASHEW RICOTTA

1. Place all the cashew ricotta ingredients in a blender and blend until creamy and smooth. Serve with the quinoa bowl, placing the lemon wedges on top.

CHUNKY SALMON MINT BURGERS

This is comfort food done in a healthy way. Despite salmon's tremendous nutritional value, I was getting a little tired of it and its very particular taste. With a little experimentation, I found that adding mint and other herbs gives the fish a whole new dimension of rich flavor.

INGREDIENTS (4 Servings):

1 pound wild-caught salmon fillets (about 2 large fillets), diced

2 tablespoons whole-grain mustard

1 handful fresh flat-leaf parsley, finely chopped

1 handful fresh mint, finely chopped

Juice of ½ lemon

¼ white onion, finely chopped

1 tablespoon extra-virgin olive oil

Sea salt and freshly ground black pepper, to taste

1 head broccoli

DIRECTIONS:

1. Preheat the oven to 425°F. Line a baking sheet with parchment paper.

2. In a large bowl, combine the salmon, mustard, parsley, mint, lemon juice, onion, and olive oil together thoroughly until it is quite sticky. Season liberally with salt and pepper.

3. Divide the mixture into 4 even parts, and form 1 burger from each quarter. Place the burgers on the prepared baking sheet, leaving plenty of space between them. Bake for about 25 minutes, or until golden and crisp.

4. Ten minutes before the burgers are done, steam the head of broccoli for 5 minutes in a steamer basket over simmering water, then chop coarsely and season to taste with salt and pepper. Serve the burgers and broccoli together and enjoy!

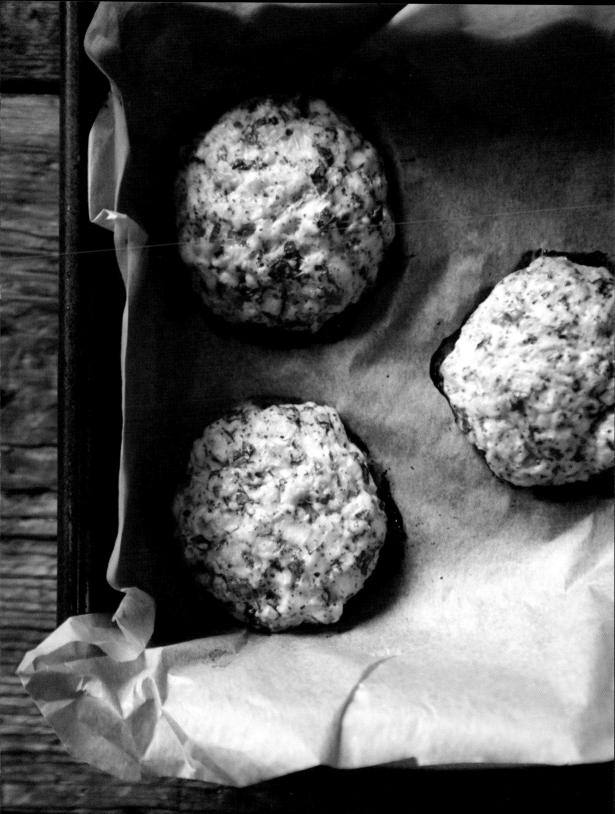

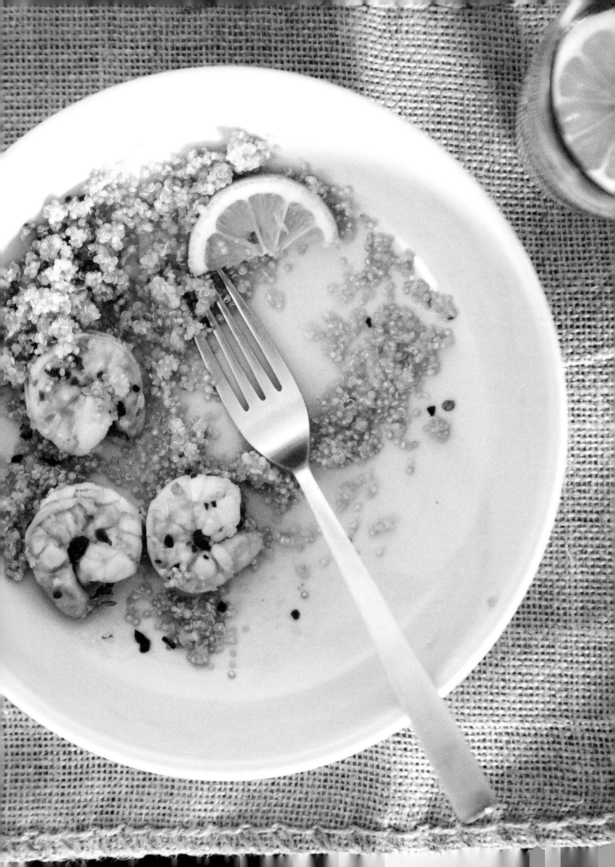

LEMON CHILI PRAWNS

I came from a landlocked country where seafood wasn't readily available. Moving abroad and tasting prawns for the first time made me realize how much I'd missed! Called *kreveta* in Czech, this dish is very simple, yet so full of flavor. Served with quinoa, it's rich in protein while the sauce is as good as a flu shot, thanks to the lemon, chili, and garlic.

INGREDIENTS (2 Servings):

Juice of 2 large lemons
3 garlic cloves, crushed
1 tablespoon extra-virgin olive oil
2 tablespoons red pepper flakes
Pinch of sea salt
Freshly ground black pepper, to taste
12–15 raw prawns
½ cup quinoa
1 cup filtered water

DIRECTIONS:

1. In a medium bowl, combine the lemon juice, garlic, olive oil, red pepper flakes, salt, and pepper.
2. Remove the prawns from their shells and wash thoroughly. Pat dry, then place in the bowl with the garlic mixture and marinate for at least 20 minutes at room temperature.
3. Rinse the quinoa well with cold water, then place it in a medium pot. Cover with the filtered water. Bring to a boil, cover, and lower the heat. Simmer on low for 12 to 15 minutes, or until the water is completely absorbed. Turn off the heat and stretch a kitchen towel over the pot, but underneath the lid, for 5 minutes.
4. While the quinoa rests, sauté the prawns with a small amount of the marinade (reserving the rest) in a large nonstick skillet over medium heat for 2 minutes per side. Once they're done, pour the rest of the marinade into the pan and let it warm up for a few seconds.
5. Top the quinoa with the cooked prawns and sauce; serve immediately.

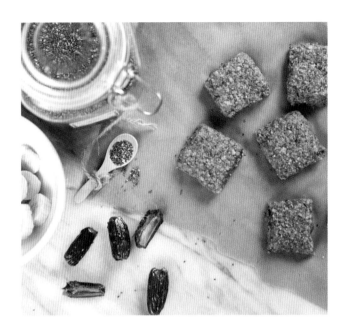

SUMMIT SNACK

There's nothing better than sitting down on top of a mountain with breathtaking views and resting your feet while you gorge on a snack that you prepared at home. These bars are also a great post-workout snack, and they travel well, too!

INGREDIENTS (10 Servings):

1½ cups raw almonds, soaked overnight in filtered water and rinsed well

¾ cup pitted Medjool dates, soaked briefly in filtered water until soft

1 banana, sliced

3 tablespoons chia seeds, soaked in 6 tablespoons filtered water until gelled

1 tablespoon ground cinnamon

1 tablespoon ground turmeric

1 tablespoon green superfood powder

½ teaspoon sea salt

DIRECTIONS:

1. Blend the almonds and dates in a blender or food processor until chunky.
2. Empty the blended mixture into a bowl, then add the banana, chia seeds, cinnamon, turmeric, green superfood powder, and salt, and mix well.
3. Press the mixture into an 8 × 8-inch dish and refrigerate until set.
4. Cut into 10 equal pieces and serve.

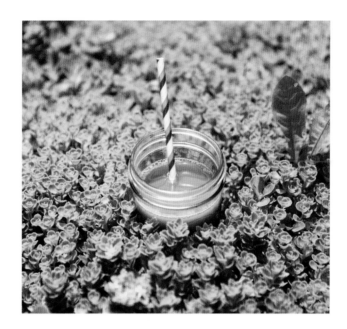

VERY GREEN JUICE

This nourishing treat is wonderful for adding a high-nutrition boost to your day. Pineapple, kale, and apples give this tasty beverage a seriously healthy punch.

INGREDIENTS (2 Servings):

1 green apple, cored but not peeled

½ bulb fennel, coarsely chopped

½ cup pineapple chunks, fresh or frozen

1 cup coarsely chopped kale

1 handful fresh thyme, leaves picked and coarsely chopped

1 teaspoon green superfood powder

½ cup filtered water

DIRECTIONS:

1. Blend all the ingredients in a blender until smooth. Strain through a fine-mesh sieve to remove the fiber.
2. Save the fiber for later snacking! I freeze it in ice pop molds for a quick and healthy snack.

SCHNITZEL WITH FENNEL SAUERKRAUT

Wiener schnitzel is a Czech classic, so once in a while I'm obliged to have it. I created this healthy version not long ago and knew I had hit the jackpot when I came home and my fiancé had finished four fillets in one sitting.

INGREDIENTS (2 Servings):

FENNEL SAUERKRAUT

½ cup almonds, soaked in filtered water for several hours, preferably overnight

2 tablespoons raw apple cider vinegar

2 garlic cloves, crushed

Juice of ½ lemon

2 tablespoons extra-virgin olive oil

Sea salt and freshly ground black pepper, to taste

1 bulb fennel, julienned

1 medium carrot, peeled and julienned

SCHNITZEL

2 free-range organic boneless, skinless chicken breasts

½ cup coconut flour

1 organic pasture-raised egg, beaten

¾ cup almond meal

Pinch of sea salt and freshly ground black pepper

3 tablespoons extra-virgin coconut oil, for frying, plus more as needed

Lemon slices, for serving

DIRECTIONS:

FENNEL SAUERKRAUT

1. Combine the almonds, apple cider vinegar, garlic, lemon juice, and olive oil in a blender. Blend until smooth, then season to taste with salt and pepper.

2. In separate bowl, combine the fennel and carrot, then pour over the almond dressing and toss to coat.

SCHNITZEL

1. Wash the chicken breasts, dry well, and cover with parchment paper. With a meat mallet or the back of a large knife, pound each breast to flatten it into a large, ½-inch-thick cutlet.

2. Set up three deep plates. Fill the first with the coconut flour, the second with the beaten egg, and the third with the almond meal. Season the coconut flour liberally with salt and pepper.

3. Dip the fillets into the coconut flour first, then the egg, then the almond meal, coating thoroughly.

4. In a large nonstick frying pan, heat the coconut oil over medium-high heat. When the oil is properly hot, sauté the fillets, cooking for approximately 3 minutes on each side. Cook the fillets one at a time, cleaning the pan with a paper towel and adding more coconut oil as you go.

5. Serve the schnitzel with a slice of lemon on top and the fennel sauerkraut on the side.

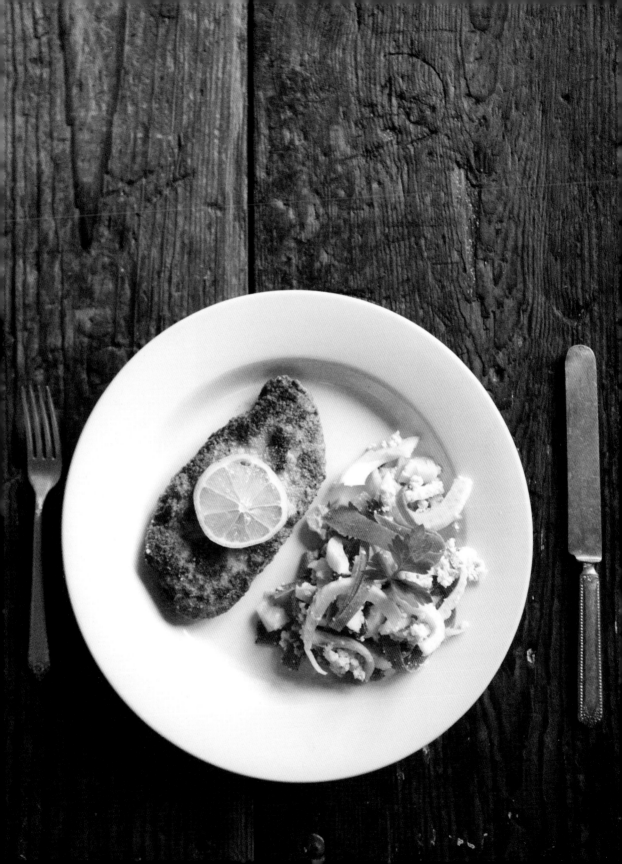

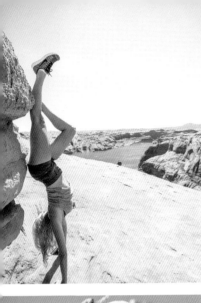
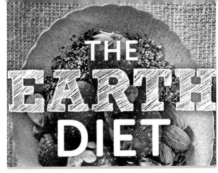
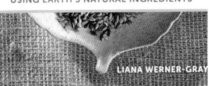

THE EARTH DIET

YOUR COMPLETE GUIDE TO LIVING USING EARTH'S NATURAL INGREDIENTS

LIANA WERNER-GRAY

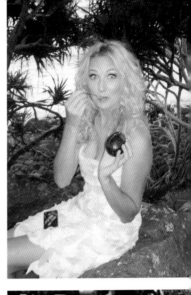
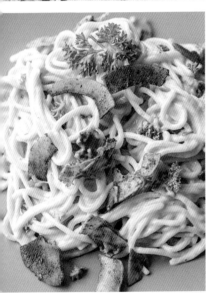
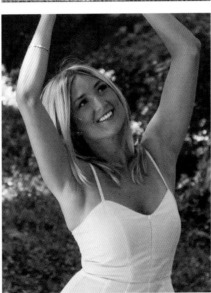
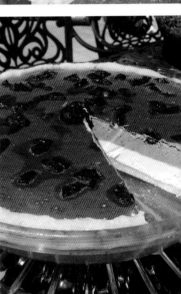
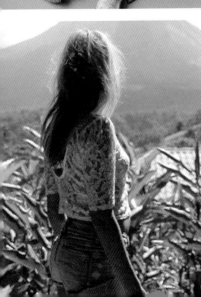
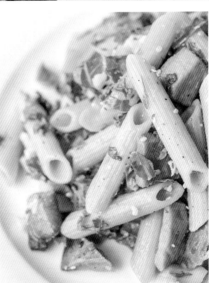
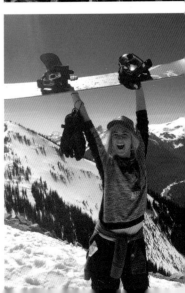

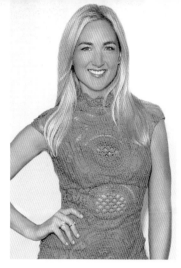

Unhealthy Foods Made Healthy

LIANA WERNER-GRAY

I have a brand-new relationship with food compared to eight years ago, before I started living "The Earth Diet Principles," which is basically just eating what Earth naturally provides. When I started relying on nature and allowed it to nourish my body every day, my old thought patterns and emotions around food also eventually transformed.

The recipes I have included here all changed my life. Making healthy versions of my favorite unhealthy foods helped me break free of my addiction to junk food. When we eat flavors we love, we are fulfilled and don't feel deprived or crave the stuff we know isn't good for us. And I was able to heal so many health issues using food, including a golf ball–size tumor in my lymphatic system, chronic fatigue, digestive problems, and binge eating. Being healthy is the best feeling in the world!

NATIONALITY: Australian

LIVES IN: New York, NY, USA

CERTIFICATIONS: Best-selling author of *The Earth Diet* and *10-Minute Recipes*, radio host, health and nutrition coach, natural foods chef

FAVORITE WAYS TO MOVE: Walking, dancing, yoga, snowboarding, wake boarding

KITCHEN MUST-HAVES: Vitamix, cumin, turmeric, Redmond Real Salt, pHresh Products cacao powder, Nutiva coconut oil

SEEN IN/KNOWN FOR: Miss Earth Australia

FIND HER ONLINE:
www.lianawernergray.com

 /theearthdiet   @lianawernergray

 /theearthdiet   /lianawernergray

EASY HOMEMADE CHIA SEED JAM

Chia seeds are surprisingly high in protein and do a great job to fill us up without feeling too full or heavy. In this jam they add health benefits plus make a delicious-looking gelatinous jam that is good as a side, snack, on toast or waffles, or with dessert! I also love to use this condiment with roast chicken, turkey, or beef.

INGREDIENTS (12 Servings):

2 cups berries of choice, diced (strawberries work well)
1 cup water
¼ cup chia seeds
¼ cup pure maple syrup or raw honey

DIRECTIONS:

1. In a large pot, combine all ingredients. Bring to a boil.
2. Reduce the heat to a simmer, stirring constantly so the chia seeds do not burn.
3. When the mixture has thickened and the fruit is entirely broken down (about 10 minutes), let cool, and then place in a glass jar. Cool completely before refrigerating.

Note: The jam is ready to eat immediately, but refrigerating it overnight improves consistency. Serve on gluten-free rolls, or use as a garnish for a special dessert!

Variations: Use one kind of berry (blueberries, blackberries, raspberries, mulberries, or cranberries), or make mixed berry jam by using ¼ cup each of strawberries, blackberries, raspberries, and blueberries.

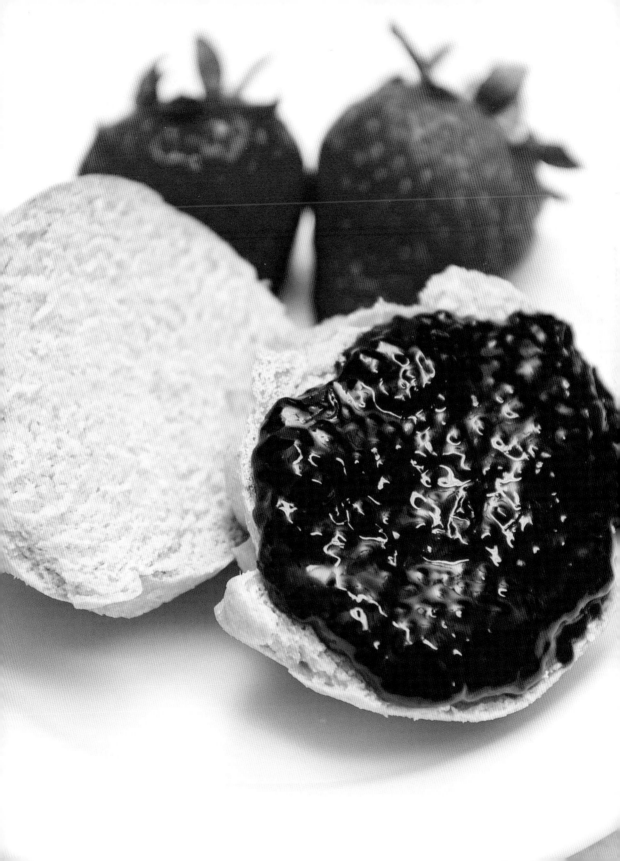

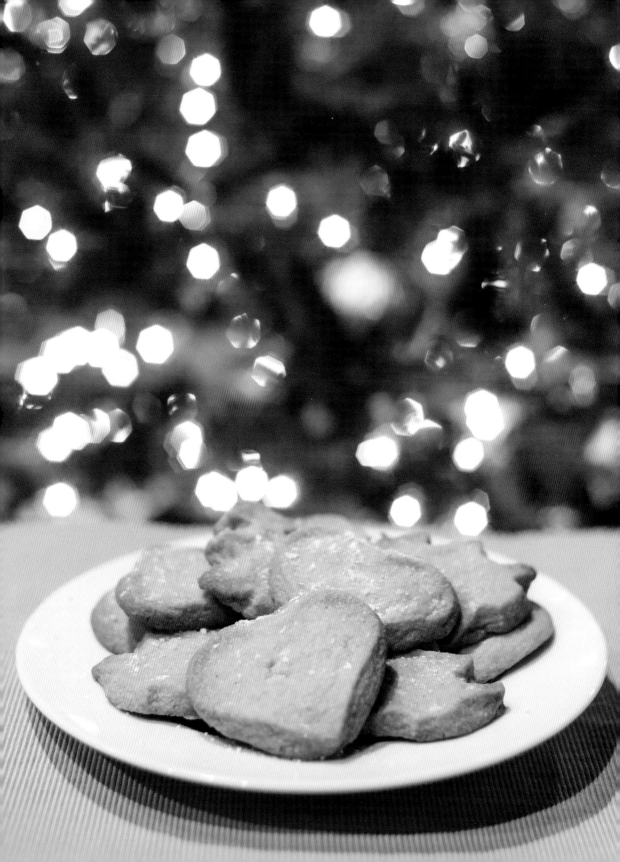

FOUR-INGREDIENT VEGAN SHORTBREAD COOKIES

This is for us—the ones who love melt-in-your-mouth, buttery shortbread but want it to be healthier than the traditional shortbread as we know it. You won't miss the butter in these delicious little bites!

INGREDIENTS (12 Cookies):

1 cup vegan shortening (such as Nutiva)
⅔ cup organic confectioner's (powdered) sugar
2 cups organic flour
⅛ teaspoon sea salt

DIRECTIONS:

1. Preheat the oven to 350°F. Line a baking sheet with parchment paper.
2. In a large mixing bowl, use a hand mixer to beat the shortening until creamy. Add the sugar and continue beating until well blended.
3. Gradually mix in the flour and salt until a soft, thick dough forms. Shape the dough into 1-inch balls and arrange on the prepared baking sheet. Use your fingers to press the dough to ¼ inch thickness (or roll out the dough on a lightly floured surface and use cookie cutters to cut into shapes).
4. Bake for 13 to 15 minutes, until golden brown.

BUFFALO CHICKEN PENNE

Ever since moving to America, I've come to love the flavor of Buffalo sauce! This classic Buffalo sauce with organic chicken and gluten-free pasta is one of my favorites! What's better than that? Maybe some cheesy flavor with nutritional yeast.

INGREDIENTS (4 Servings):

1 (8-ounce) box red lentil penne

⅔ cup hot sauce

½ cup plus 1 tablespoon extra-virgin coconut oil, melted, divided

1 tablespoon MCT oil

1 tablespoon raw honey

1 tablespoon apple cider vinegar

1 tablespoon sweet paprika

½ teaspoon garlic powder

¼ teaspoon sea salt

1 pound boneless, skinless organic chicken, cubed

DIRECTIONS:

1. In a large pot, prepare the penne according to the package directions. Drain and set aside.

2. Meanwhile, in a large bowl, combine the hot sauce, ½ cup of the coconut oil, MCT oil, honey, apple cider vinegar, paprika, garlic, and salt. Stir until a thick sauce forms.

3. In a separate bowl, combine the chicken and half of the sauce. Set aside to marinate for a few minutes.

4. Heat a large skillet with the remaining 1 tablespoon coconut oil. Add the chicken and cook, stirring occasionally, until cooked through, about 8 minutes.

5. Add the drained pasta and remaining sauce to the chicken. Stir to combine and serve immediately.

Make it vegan: Replace the chicken with 1 large head of cauliflower cut into florets. Bake the cauliflower at 350°F for 20 minutes, or pan-fry it.

Make it "cheezy": Add 3 tablespoons nutritional yeast to the sauce mixture for a vegan-friendly "cheeze sauce."

Note: I use Nutiva butter-flavored coconut oil in this recipe to make it extra buttery.

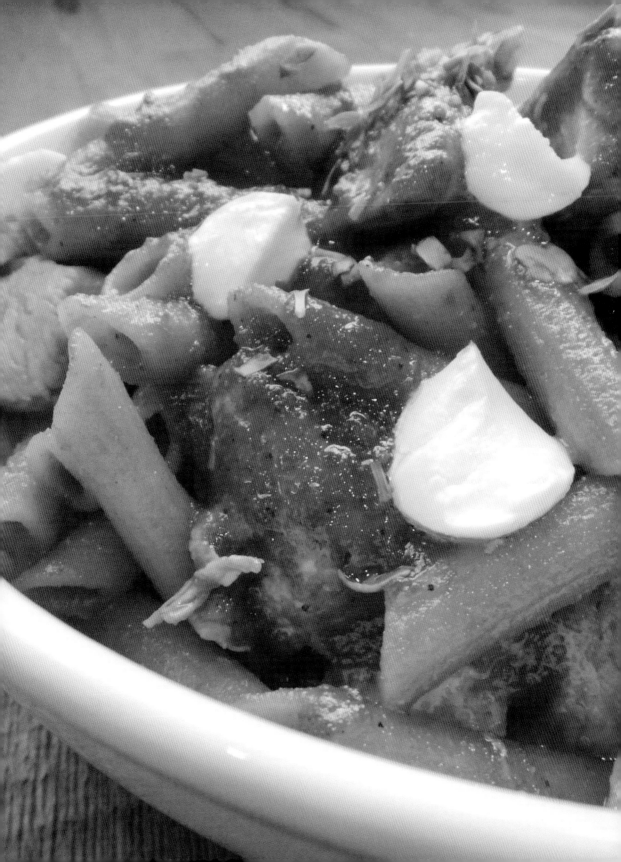

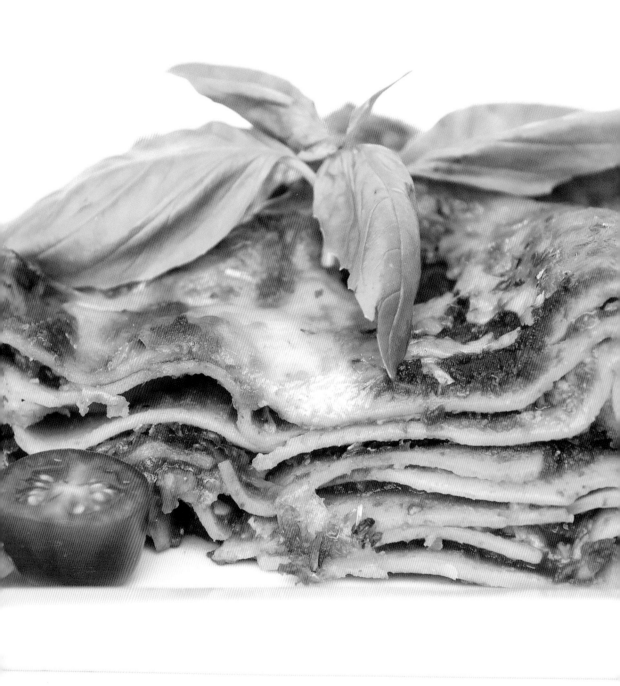

GLUTEN-FREE LASAGNA

Lasagna is a classic staple that I can't live without! The green lentil lasagna sheets in this version are gluten-free and high in protein. This super simple recipe, with just three layers of the pasta sheets, tomato sauce, and cheese, is a great base to launch your creativity. And if you are busy, make up a batch on Sunday, freeze or refrigerate it, and you can enjoy lasagna throughout the week.

INGREDIENTS (4 Servings):

1 (25-ounce) jar organic pasta sauce (or 3 cups homemade)

1 (7.05-ounce) box green lentil lasagna noodles (such as Explore Cuisine)

1 recipe Cashew Ricotta (page 145) or 1 cup plant-based or dairy mozzarella

½ teaspoon garlic salt

1 tablespoon dried oregano

1 tablespoon dried basil

1 tablespoon dried thyme

1 tablespoon dried parsley

DIRECTIONS:

1. Preheat the oven to 400°F.
2. Coat the bottom of a 9 × 13-inch pan with sauce. Place a layer of lasagna sheets over the sauce and top with more sauce. Sprinkle on one-third of the ricotta. Combine all of the spices in a small bowl, then sprinkle one-third of the mixture on top of the ricotta.
3. Add two more layers of lasagna noodles, sauce, cheese, and spices.
4. Bake for 40 minutes, or until the top is golden brown. Let sit for 5 to 10 minutes before serving.

CASHEW CREAM BITES WITH CHOCOLATE SAUCE

Ice cream lovers, you must try this recipe. It's a totally guilt-free ice cream made with cashews and just loaded with nutrition: vitamins C and E, good omega fats, protein, and antioxidants. Together with the chocolate sauce, it delivers a mind-blowing explosion of nutritious flavor. If you like bonbon ice cream with vanilla on the bottom and chocolate on top, you are going to enjoy this! This might be one of the recipes I've made the most. Be sure to whip the mixture thoroughly in the blender so it is super creamy.

INGREDIENTS (15 Servings):

CASHEW ICE CREAM BITES

1½ cups cashews, soaked in water for 4 hours and drained
Juice of 1 small lemon
½ cup pure maple syrup
¼ cup extra-virgin coconut oil
1 tablespoon pure vanilla extract
2 teaspoons maca powder
Pinch of sea salt

CHOCOLATE SAUCE

⅔ cup cacao powder
½ cup pure maple syrup
¼ cup extra-virgin coconut oil, melted

DIRECTIONS:

CASHEW CREAM BITES

1. Blend the cashews, lemon juice, maple syrup, coconut oil, vanilla, maca powder, and salt in a high-speed blender until smooth. There should be absolutely no lumps!
2. Scoop the mixture into the cups of a mini-muffin tin and place in the freezer for 5 minutes.

CHOCOLATE SAUCE

1. Blend the cacao powder, maple syrup, and melted coconut oil in a blender until smooth, thick, and creamy.
2. Add a spoonful of chocolate sauce to each cashew cream bite. Serve immediately, or store in the freezer to set the chocolate.

"Food is so powerful, and everything we put into our body literally will become our body—it becomes our cells, our bones, our nervous system, and our blood. This is why it is crucial to put only high-quality, beautiful, natural foods into our temple."

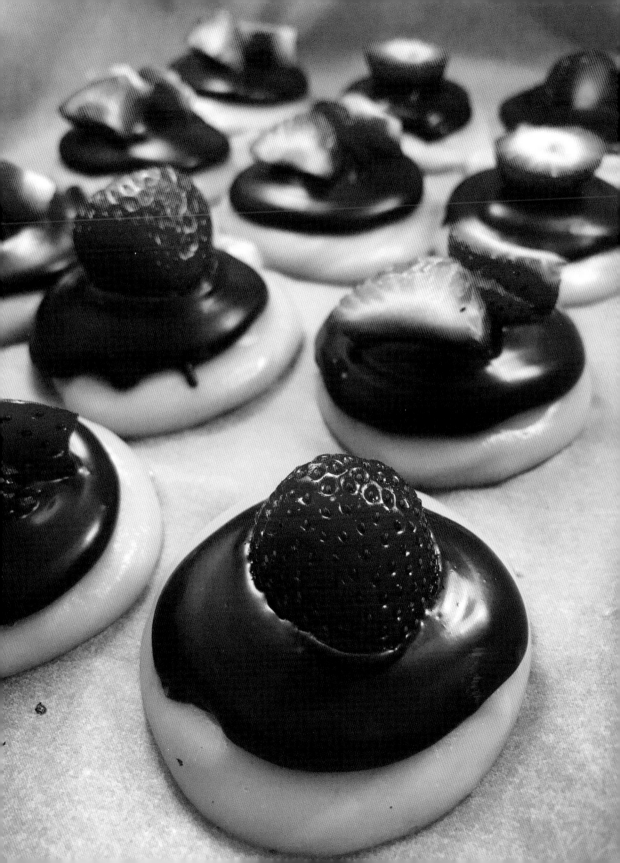

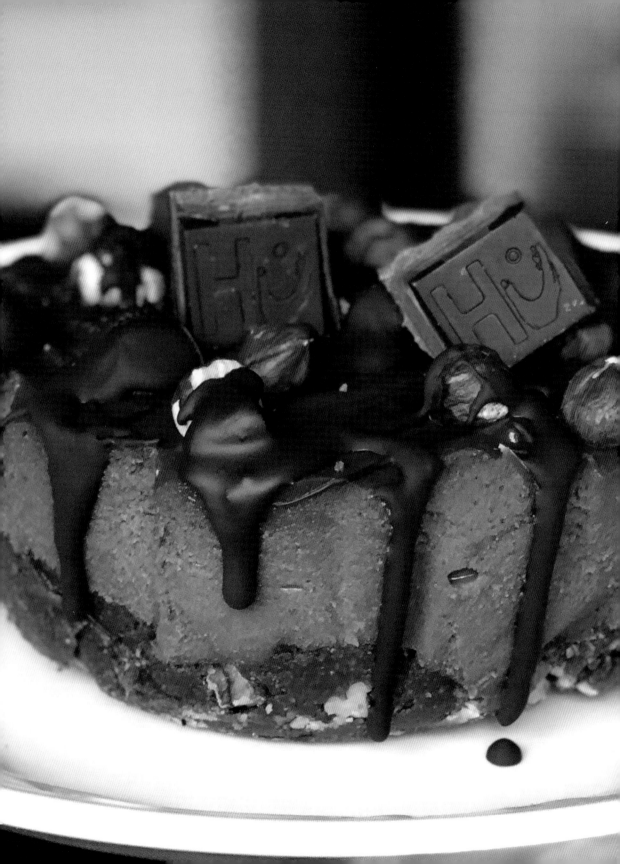

CHOCOLATE HAZELNUT CHEESECAKE

This cheesecake is a dream come true—I literally dreamed of this and then created the recipe, and here it is! If you love a combo of smooth chocolate, creamy cheesecake, and whole toasted hazelnuts, you will absolutely love this recipe! Plan ahead when you want to make this cheesecake. You'll need 4 hours to soak the nuts and 4 hours of freezing time, but only 25 minutes of hands-on time to make this decadent dessert.

INGREDIENTS (16 Servings):

BASE

2 cups almond meal

2 cups hazelnut meal

4 tablespoons cacao powder

1 tablespoon MCT oil

5 Medjool dates, pitted

5 tablespoons pure maple syrup or raw honey

FILLING

1½ cups cashews, soaked in water for 4 hours and drained

1½ cups hazelnuts, soaked in water for 4 hours and drained

¾ cup plus 2 tablespoons pure maple syrup

½ cup lemon juice (approximately 2 large lemons)

½ cup refined coconut oil

¼ cup MCT oil

3 tablespoons cacao powder

1 tablespoon pure vanilla extract

⅛ teaspoon sea salt

TOPPING

¼–½ cup hazelnuts

1 (2-ounce) vegan dark chocolate hazelnut bar (such as Hu Kitchen)

DIRECTIONS:

BASE

1. Pulse the almond meal, hazelnut meal, cacao powder, MCT oil, dates, and maple syrup in a food processor until well combined. (Or mash the dates and combine all the ingredients with your hands.) The mixture should be just moist enough to hold together.
2. Press the mixture evenly into a deep-dish pie plate or springform pan (large enough to hold 2½ quarts), to cover the bottom and sides of the dish. Set aside.

FILLING

1. Blend the cashews, hazelnuts, maple syrup, lemon juice, coconut oil, MCT oil, cacao powder, vanilla, and salt in a high-speed blender until the mixture is very smooth and light in texture. There should be no chunks. Pour the filling into the crust.

TOPPING

1. Evenly distribute the whole hazelnuts on top of the filling. Melt the dark chocolate hazelnut bar in a small saucepan over low heat, then drizzle it over the cheesecake.
2. Freeze for 4 hours. Once set, cut into slices and serve. Well wrapped, this will keep in the refrigerator for up to 2 weeks.

RAW CHERRY "CHEESECAKE" WITH ALMOND CRUST

This heavenly vanilla cheesecake topped with a beautiful layer of cherry cheesecake makes me feel like I'm in Paris when eating it! This recipe is super packed with antioxidants and high in protein!

INGREDIENTS (16 Servings):

CRUST
4 cups raw almonds
5 tablespoons pure maple syrup
Pinch of sea salt

CHEESECAKE LAYER
1½ cups cashews, soaked in water for 3 hours and drained
¼ cup plus 2 tablespoons pure maple syrup (or raw honey if not vegan)
¼ cup plus 2 tablespoons extra-virgin coconut oil
⅓ cup lemon juice
1½ teaspoons pure vanilla extract
Pinch of sea salt

CHERRY LAYER
1½ cups cashews, soaked in water for 3 hours and drained
2 cups cherries, pitted, plus more for garnish (optional)
¼ cup plus 2 tablespoons pure maple syrup (or raw honey if not vegan)
¼ cup plus 2 tablespoons extra-virgin coconut oil
¼ cup lemon juice
1½ teaspoons pure vanilla extract
Pinch of sea salt

DIRECTIONS:

CRUST
1. Grind the almonds into a fine meal in a food processor. Stir in the syrup and salt, adding a little water if needed to create a moist mixture. Press the filling into a 9-inch deep-dish pie plate, covering the bottom and sides.

CHEESECAKE LAYER
1. Blend the cashews, maple syrup, coconut oil, lemon juice, vanilla, and salt in a high-speed blender until smooth. Pour into the crust and freeze while preparing the cherry layer.

CHERRY LAYER
1. Blend the cashews, cherries, maple syrup, coconut oil, lemon juice, vanilla, and salt in a high-speed blender until smooth. Pour over the cheesecake layer. Arrange fresh cherries on top for garnish, if desired.
2. Freeze for 4 hours or overnight before serving.

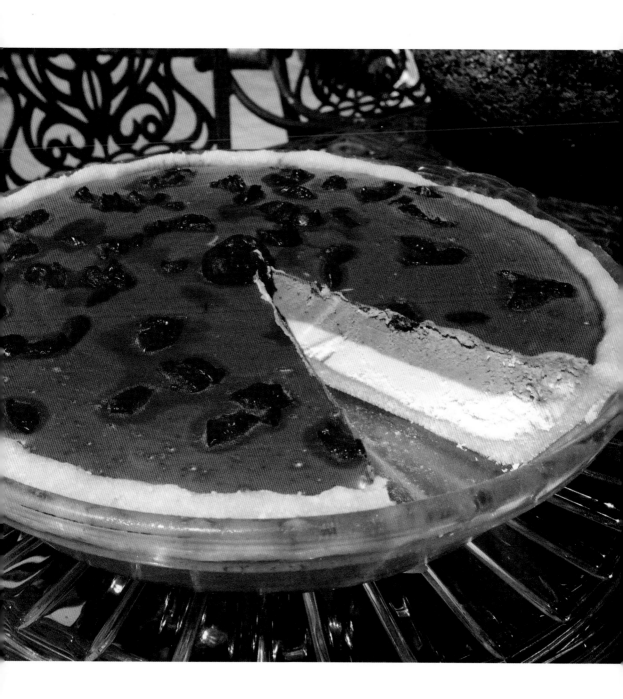

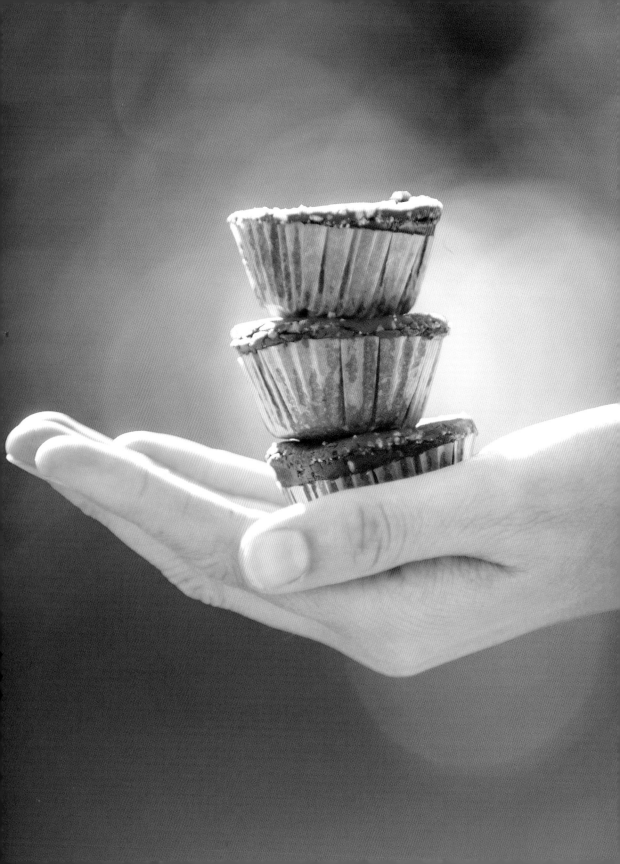

CHOCOLATE SUNFLOWER BUTTER CUPS

There are so many health benefits in chocolate; cacao is the ingredient in chocolate that makes it healthy, and these little cups are as tasty as they are nutritious. A handful of sunflower seeds will take care of your hunger, while also supplying significant amounts of vitamin E, magnesium, and selenium.

INGREDIENTS (12 Servings):

¾ cup cacao butter

2–6 tablespoons cacao powder

½ cup almond meal

3 tablespoons pure maple syrup

1 cup sunflower butter

DIRECTIONS:

1. Melt the cacao butter in a small saucepan over very low heat. Once melted, add the cacao powder, almond meal, and maple syrup and mix well. Taste it, and then add more cacao powder if you like it darker and more maple syrup if you like it sweeter.

2. Line the cups of a mini-muffin tin with paper liners (or use mini silicone baking cups). Spoon half of the chocolate mixture into the cups, filling each one-third of the way. Reserve the other half of the mixture for the top of the cups. Put the baking cups in the freezer for 5 minutes to set.

3. Remove the cups from the freezer and add a spoonful of sunflower butter to each one. Each cup should now be two-thirds full.

4. Pour the remainder of the chocolate mixture on top of the sunflower butter. Place the cups in the freezer again, and allow them to set for 15 minutes before enjoying.

SUNFLOWER BUTTER CRISPY RICE TREATS

This is an organic spin on the traditional crispy rice treats with organic marshmallows and sunflower seed butter, which is a great nut-free alternative to creamy peanut butter. This recipe makes perfectly formed squares to take to lunch or for a quick snack from the refrigerator. It's also a great treat to bring to a party or an event!

INGREDIENTS (12 Servings):

½ cup coconut oil (such as Nutiva buttery coconut oil)

4 cups gluten-free vegan marshmallows

½ cup organic sunflower butter

¼ teaspoon pure vanilla extract

⅛ teaspoon sea salt

6 cups gluten-free crispy rice cereal

1½ cups organic chocolate chips (such as Enjoy Life)

DIRECTIONS:

1. Combine the coconut oil and marshmallows in a large, heavy pot over low heat and stir until melted.
2. Stir in the sunflower butter, vanilla, and salt, then add the cereal and mix until well combined.
3. Line a 9 × 12-inch baking dish with parchment paper, and press the rice cereal mixture into the pan.
4. Melt the chocolate chips in a small saucepan over low heat. Pour over the rice cereal mixture, then refrigerate until the chocolate is solid before serving.

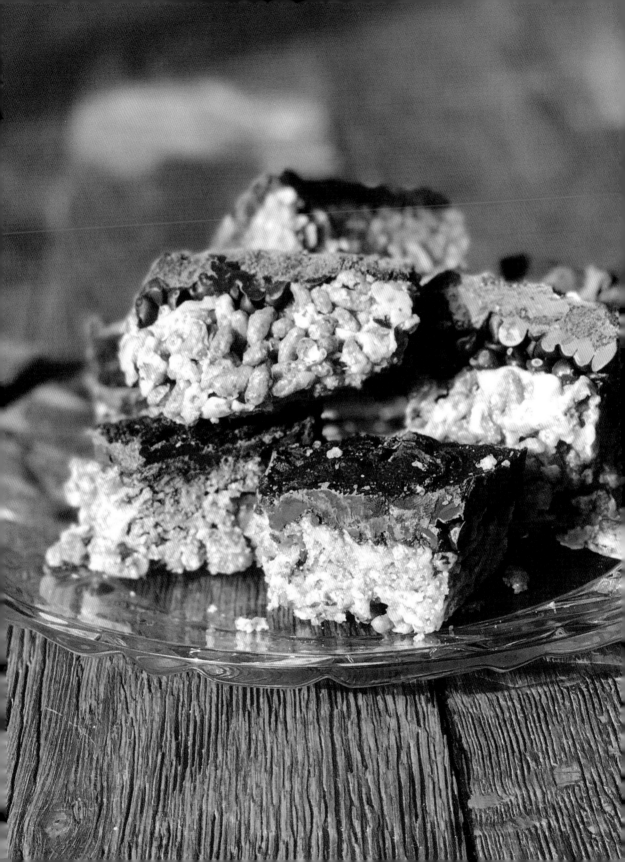

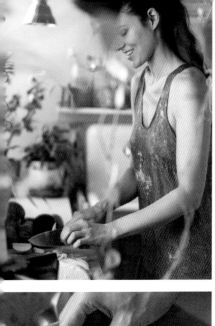
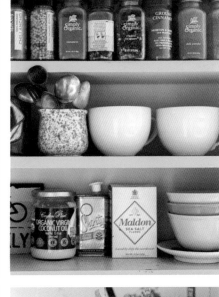
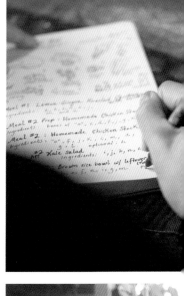
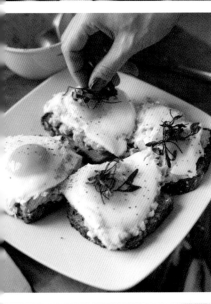
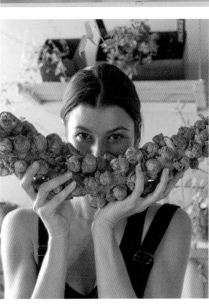
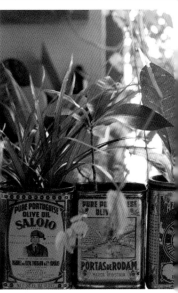
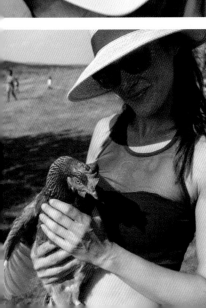
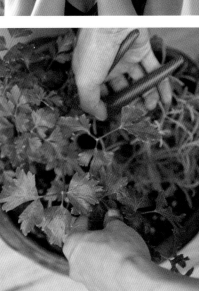
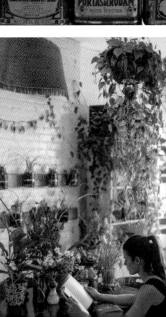

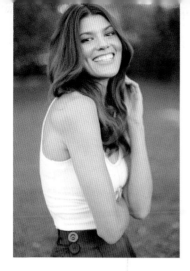

Mostly Plants

SUMMER RAYNE OAKES

I was excited to share my ideas of bringing sustainable practices to an industry that seemed devoid of that value set. The agents listened to my big-picture plans, and at the end, one of them looked me squarely in the face and said, "Well, you know 80 percent of the jobs won't be available to you because your hips are two inches too big?"

I laughed. The less obvious path is often the hardest. It's also the one, however, that reaps the greatest rewards. It is your intelligence, your resolve, your character—your whole beauty— that distinguishes you. Don't shrink because it's what you think the world wants from you. We need not be bystanders or passive players in this game.

NATIONALITY: American

LIVES IN: Brooklyn, NY, USA

CERTIFICATIONS/DEGREES: B.S. in Environmental Science and Entomology from Cornell University, Certified Holistic Nutritionist

FAVORITE WAYS TO MOVE: Yoga, boxing, meditation, dancing, hiking

KITCHEN MUST-HAVES: Cutting board scraper, good chef's knife, cardamom, home-grown herbs

SEEN IN/KNOWN FOR: Pirelli Calendar, Levi Strauss, Aveeno, Toyota Prius C, Modo Summer Rayne Oakes Eco Eyewear, Portico Home

FIND HER ONLINE:
www.sugardetox.me
www.homesteadbrooklyn.com

@sroakes   @sugardetoxme

@homesteadbrooklyn   /summerrayneoakes

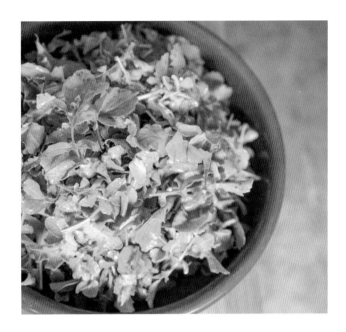

ARUGULA SALAD

The best salads are kept simple. If you have the freshest ingredients, like this fresh-from-the-farm arugula, all you need is a spritz of lemon, olive oil, and a little sea salt and pepper.

INGREDIENTS (2 Servings):

4 ounces arugula

Juice of 1 lemon

1 tablespoon extra-virgin olive oil

Sea salt and freshly ground black pepper, to taste

DIRECTIONS:

1. Place the arugula in a bowl. Juice the lemon over the arugula, then add olive oil, salt, and pepper.

2. Gently toss and enjoy.

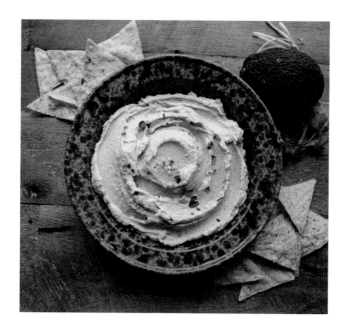

AVOCADO HUMMUS

I was inspired to make this avocado hummus by Joy the Baker's blog. Don't peel the chickpeas, and add cumin, red pepper, and extra garlic for added flavor. For even more zing, add half a jalapeño pepper. Serve with baked tortilla chips or sweet potato chips.

INGREDIENTS (6 Servings):

1 (14-ounce) can chickpeas, rinsed and drained

2 ripe avocados, peeled, pitted, and cut into chunks

½ cup extra-virgin olive oil, plus more for serving

¼ cup freshly squeezed lemon juice, plus more as needed

3 tablespoons tahini

3 garlic cloves, crushed

½ teaspoon ground cumin

½ jalapeño pepper, seeded and chopped (optional)

Sea salt and freshly ground black pepper, to taste

½ teaspoon red pepper flakes, for serving

DIRECTIONS:

1. Blend the chickpeas, avocados, olive oil, lemon juice, tahini, garlic, cumin, and jalapeño (if using) in a food processor. Add more lemon juice, if needed, for smoother texture.

2. Drizzle with olive oil, season with salt and pepper, and sprinkle with red pepper flakes.

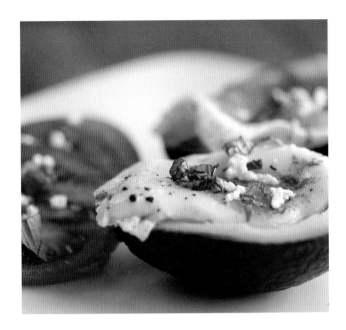

SUNNY-SIDE-UP EGGS IN AN AVOCADO

I love the idea of having a "pocket" of food. Give me a good lettuce wrap, a deviled egg, or even an endive boat on any given day. This recipe is, in a way, a breakfast "pocket"—using an avocado half as a bed for a drippy, yolky egg.

INGREDIENTS (2 Servings):

1 tablespoon extra-virgin olive oil
2 medium organic pasture-raised eggs
Sea salt and freshly ground black pepper, to taste
1 avocado, halved
¼ heirloom tomato, sliced
Ground cumin, to taste
4–7 basil leaves, chiffonade cut
Crumble of goat cheese feta, for serving

DIRECTIONS:

1. Heat the olive oil in a skillet over medium heat. Crack the eggs into the pan, season with salt and pepper, and cover for 2 to 3 minutes. Cook to your preference.

2. While the eggs are cooking, slice open an avocado, remove the pit, and spoon out 1 to 2 tablespoons so that an egg can fit into the hollow. Put tomato slices on the side of a plate.

3. Remove each egg with a solid metal spatula and place it gently into an avocado half. Season with more salt, pepper, and cumin.

4. Top the eggs and tomato with basil, crumble a little goat cheese feta on top, and enjoy!

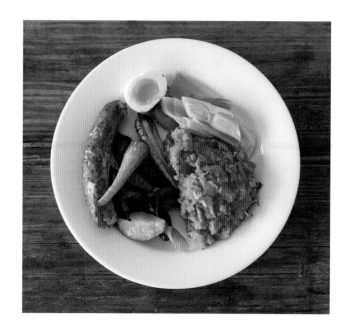

MOROCCAN CARROT MASH

One of the wonderful bonuses of being part of the local food scene is access to the freshest ingredients from local farmers and food makers. This carrot mash with harissa (Moroccan red chile paste) was introduced to me by Chef Audrey Snyder. If you're not keen on making your own red chile paste, Mina Harissa sells a delicious one that's made without any sugar.

INGREDIENTS (4 Servings):

1 tablespoon extra-virgin olive oil
1 tablespoon grass-fed ghee
10 large carrots, peeled and cut into ¾-inch pieces
1 cup vegetable stock
Sea salt, to taste
Grated orange or lemon zest
2 garlic cloves, crushed
2 teaspoons harissa
1 tablespoon lemon juice
Freshly ground black pepper, to taste
1 handful of fresh flat-leaf parsley, coarsely chopped
Pistachios, chopped, for serving

DIRECTIONS:

1. Heat the olive oil and ghee in a large skillet over medium-high heat. Add the carrots and sauté for 5 to 7 minutes, stirring often. Let them soften.
2. Add the vegetable stock. Turn the heat to medium-low, cover the pan, and cook for another 25 minutes, until the carrots are soft and there is hardly any liquid left.
3. Transfer the carrots to a food processor, add salt, and pulse to a paste.
4. Let cool, then add the orange zest, garlic, harissa, lemon juice, and some pepper. Stir and serve topped with parsley and pistachios.

CHARRED CAULIFLOWER, PEPPERS, AND EGG

Leftovers are a terrible thing to waste—so I turned a leftover charred cauliflower and shishito pepper dish into a delicious side, along with some leftover beef, a sunny-side-up egg, and half of a ripe, juicy blood orange. I swear by Maldon salt, so if you have some on hand, give it a try.

INGREDIENTS (4 Servings):

1 head cauliflower, trimmed, halved, and cut into 1½-inch wedges

3 tablespoons extra-virgin olive oil, divided

Sea salt and freshly ground black pepper, to taste

8 garlic cloves, roughly chopped

1 tablespoon avocado oil

12 shishito peppers

½ cup whole almonds, toasted and roughly chopped

1 cup plus 1 tablespoon roughly chopped fresh flat-leaf parsley, divided

1 tablespoon finely grated dark chocolate

2 teaspoons sherry vinegar

DIRECTIONS:

1. Preheat the broiler. Arrange the cauliflower in a single layer on a rimmed baking sheet. Brush both sides with 2 tablespoons of the olive oil and season with salt and pepper. Broil, flipping once, until charred and tender, about 15 minutes.

2. Meanwhile, heat the remaining 1 tablespoon olive oil and the garlic in a medium skillet over medium heat. Cook until the garlic is golden, 4 to 6 minutes, then transfer the garlic and oil to a bowl and let cool.

3. Wipe the skillet clean and heat the avocado oil over medium-high heat; fry the peppers until blistered and slightly crisp, 4 to 6 minutes. Transfer the peppers to paper towels to drain; season with salt.

4. Stir the almonds, 1 cup of the parsley, chocolate, and sherry vinegar into the reserved garlic oil; spread onto a serving platter and season with salt and pepper. Top with the cauliflower; garnish with the fried peppers and remaining 1 tablespoon parsley, and serve immediately.

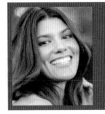

"I usually cook no-fuss, uncomplicated meals, and I try to stay away from added sugars and processed foods. Eating healthy fuels me so I can do more important adventures and ventures in life. Taking care of your body, spirit, and mind means more opportunity for you to do something amazing in the world. So make the most of it!"

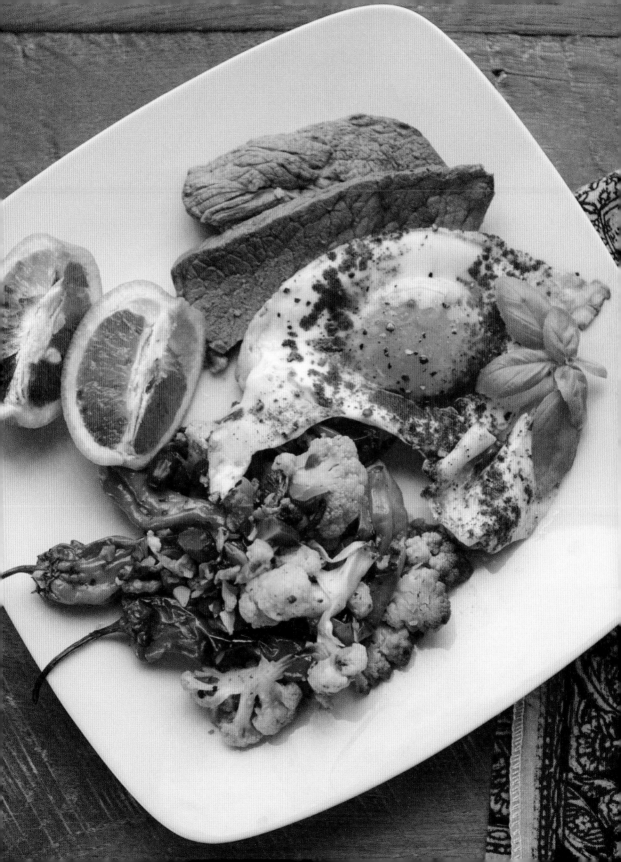

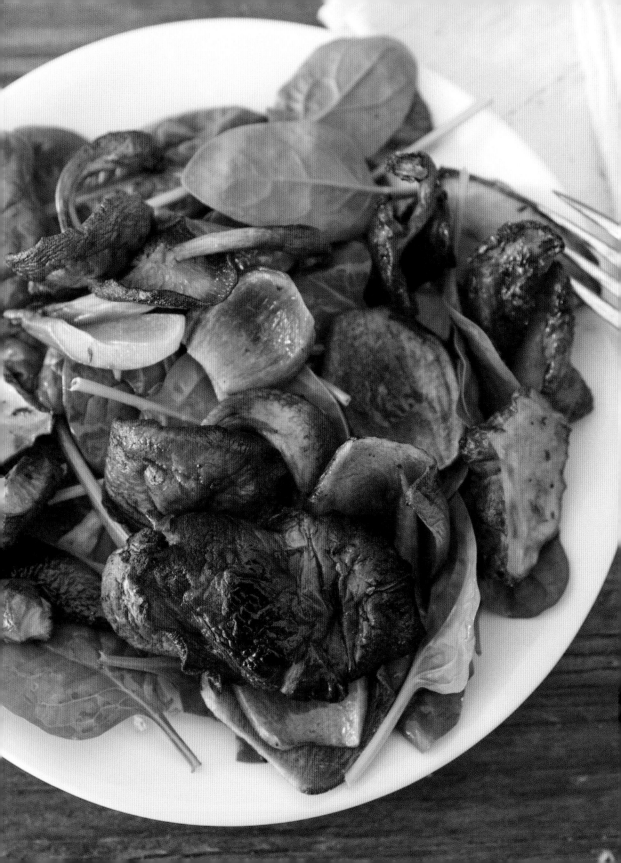

SHIITAKE, ONION, AND SUNCHOKE SALAD

Here's another fine recipe that I learned from my friend, Chef Audrey Snyder. This is a wholesome salad with the buttery crispness of sunchokes and the earthy flavor of shiitakes.

INGREDIENTS (2 Servings):

8 ounces sunchokes (Jerusalem artichokes)

4 tablespoons extra-virgin olive oil, divided

Sea salt and freshly ground black pepper, to taste

1 large red onion, quartered

8 ounces whole fresh shiitake mushrooms (stemmed if desired)

1 to 2 tablespoons water

4 ounces spinach

DIRECTIONS:

1. Preheat the oven to 350°F.
2. Scrub the sunchokes and cut out any eyes, then cut them in half. Toss with 1 tablespoon of the olive oil and a generous pinch of salt in a large bowl, then arrange the sunchoke pieces on a rimmed baking sheet. Transfer to the oven and roast for 35 to 40 minutes.
3. Heat 2 tablespoons of the remaining olive oil in a skillet over medium heat. Add the onion and cook, stirring occasionally, for about 5 minutes. Keep them in the pan if you like them more caramelized, or remove them if not. Add the mushrooms and continue to cook, tossing occasionally, until tender and lightly browned, about 8 minutes. Add the water to the skillet to give some moisture to the mushrooms. Reduce the heat to low, cover, and let steam for about 2 minutes longer.
4. Toss the sunchokes, onions, and mushrooms together in a large bowl. Next, dress the spinach with the remaining 1 tablespoon olive oil and season with salt and pepper. Top with the sunchoke and shiitake mixture and serve immediately.

MUSTARD AND MICROGREEN BEET SALAD

Salads are a girl's "no-fuss meal." They're easy to prepare, but it's nice to switch it up a bit by adding some color and whole fruit. Admittedly, sometimes I pick my veggies and fruit based on color alone, knowing that my meal will look so much more appetizing when it has a fuller spectrum of plant life.

INGREDIENTS (2 Servings):

SALAD

1 cup microgreens

1 cup wild mustard greens

1 handful raspberries

1 hard-boiled egg, peeled and quartered

1 Chioggia beet, peeled and julienned

⅓ cup chopped walnuts

DRESSING

2 tablespoons sherry vinegar

3–4 raspberries

1 tablespoon extra-virgin olive oil

Sea salt and freshly ground black pepper, to taste

DIRECTIONS:

1. Place all the salad ingredients in a bowl.
2. Put the dressing ingredients in a mason jar. Close tightly, shake vigorously, and pour over the salad.

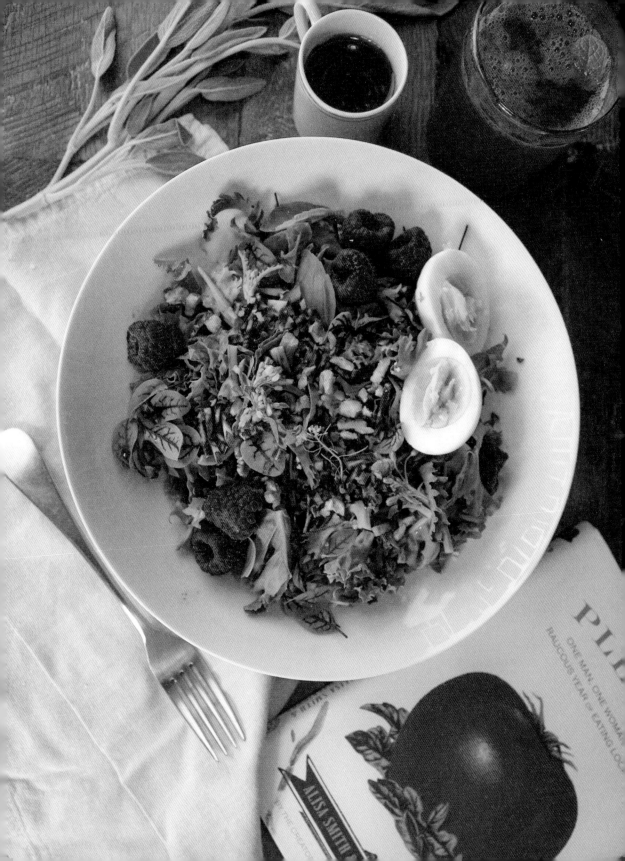

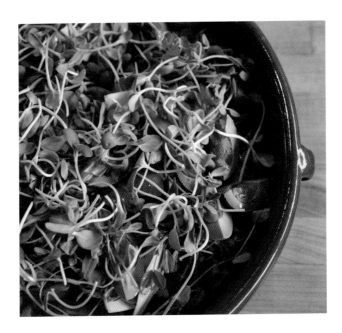

PICKLED EGG, BEET, AND PEA TENDRIL SALAD

There's a touch of whimsy to this salad, thanks to the Chioggia beets (also known as candy cane beets) and beet-dyed hard-boiled eggs.

INGREDIENTS (4 Servings):

6 hard-boiled eggs, peeled
1 (15-ounce) can pickled or canned beets
1 pound pea tendrils (or other microgreens)
3 Chioggia beets, peeled and sliced thinly
Juice of 1 lemon
2 tablespoons extra-virgin olive oil
Sea salt and freshly ground black pepper, to taste

DIRECTIONS:

1. Place the hard-boiled eggs in a glass bowl and add the pickled beets. Refrigerate for 24 to 36 hours.
2. Slice the eggs into quarters. Add to a large bowl with the pea tendrils and Chioggia beets.
3. Dress with the lemon juice, olive oil, and salt and pepper to taste, and serve immediately.

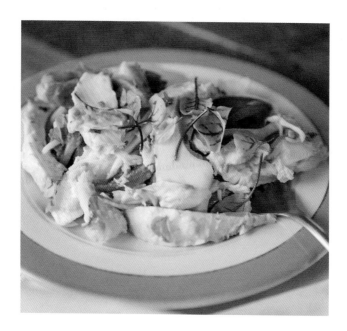

AVOCADO, TOMATO, AND CRAB SALAD

When I was a young girl, my parents would occasionally treat the family to some succulent crabmeat, which I still always find a true delight. There is a subtle sweetness to the pink meat, and when it's fresh, there is not much else that can compare.

INGREDIENTS (2 Servings):

3 king crab legs
2 avocados, peeled, pitted, and sliced
2 small heirloom tomatoes, sliced into eighths
2 ounces red-veined sorrel
1 tablespoon extra-virgin olive oil
1 lemon wedge
Sea salt and freshly ground black pepper, to taste

DIRECTIONS:

1. To prepare the crab legs, set a steamer tray in a large pot and pour 1 to 2 inches of water inside. Bring to a boil, then place the crab legs in the steamer. Cover the pot and steam for 5 minutes.

2. Remove the crab legs and crack the shells. Using a fork, remove the meat and let cool.

3. Place the avocado slices, tomatoes, and crab on a plate. Dress with the red-veined sorrel, olive oil, and a wedge of lemon, and season to taste with salt and pepper.

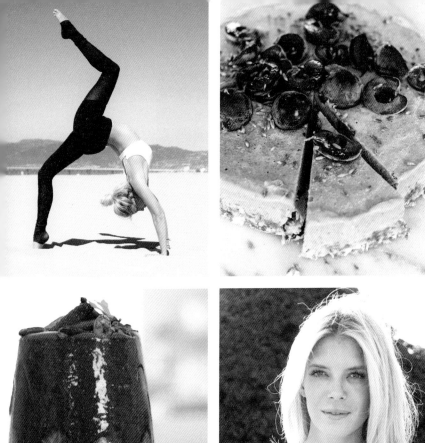
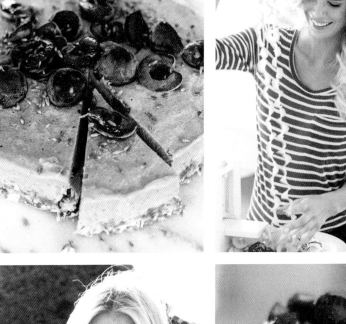
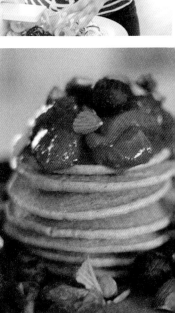
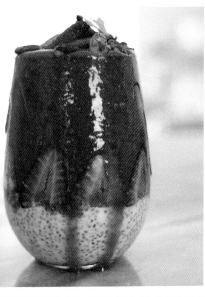
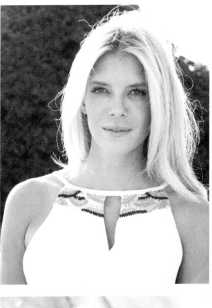
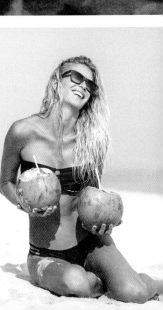
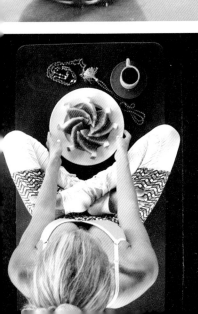
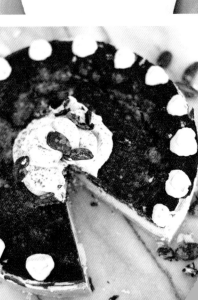

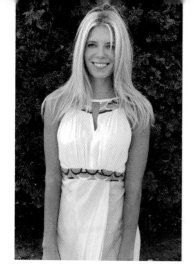

Sweets and Treats

NIKKI SHARP

I decided not to model full time until I graduated university, so at twenty-one I began my overseas career. In ten years, I went from not eating much of anything and being absolutely terrified of food and gaining weight to the complete opposite and bingeing because an agency told me to gain weight.

I needed to get healthy because I was unhappy and unfulfilled by modeling. I began learning about nutrition and yoga, and trained for a triathlon. It was then that I realized I had this huge passion for nutritious food and eating well.

Since my modeling days, I've created a successful lifestyle brand under my own name, The 5-Day Detox, which became a best-selling book and number-one app, and I most recently released my newest book, *Meal Prep Your Way to Weight Loss*. Now I love teaching others about health!

NATIONALITY: American/English

LIVES IN: Los Angeles, CA, USA

CERTIFICATIONS: Institute for Integrative Nutrition, Raw Foods and Sports Nutrition from the Institute of Optimum Nutrition (London)

FAVORITE WAYS TO MOVE: Yoga, running, hiking, plyometrics, weights, cycling

KITCHEN MUST-HAVES: Vitamix, turmeric, cayenne pepper, cinnamon

SEEN IN/KNOWN FOR: *Access Hollywood, Good Day LA, Hollywood Today Live, Extra! TV, Daily Mail*, Mind Body Green, *Men's Health, Elle*

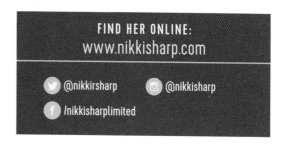

FIND HER ONLINE:
www.nikkisharp.com

@nikkirsharp   @nikkisharp

/nikkisharplimited

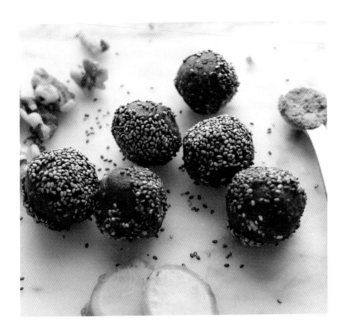

GINGERLICIOUS BLISS

These bliss balls can be eaten any time of day. They contain ginger, which is anti-inflammatory and reduces pain in the body, as well as chia seeds, which provide calcium and omega-3 fatty acids.

INGREDIENTS (20 Servings):

1 cup walnuts

¾ cup Medjool dates, pitted

2 small chunks fresh ginger, peeled

½ teaspoon pure vanilla extract

½ teaspoon ground ginger

2 tablespoons chia seeds

DIRECTIONS:

1. Combine the walnuts, dates, ginger, vanilla extract, and ground ginger in a food processor and blend well.
2. Roll the mixture into ½- to 1-inch balls, then roll the balls in chia seeds. Freeze for 1 hour before serving.

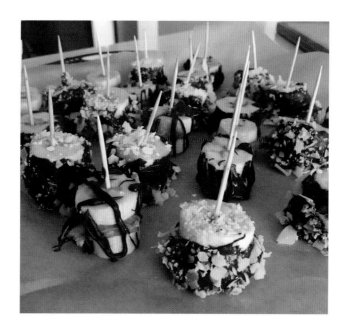

P.B. BANANA BITES

Bananas are high in potassium and a great snack! I like them with organic peanut butter and dark chocolate for a healthy treat.

INGREDIENTS (25 Servings):

4 bananas, sliced

¼ cup organic peanut butter

¼ cup dark chocolate chips

2–3 tablespoons unsweetened coconut flakes

DIRECTIONS:

1. Line a baking sheet with parchment or wax paper and lay half the banana slices on it.
2. Spread some peanut butter on each banana slice, then top with a second banana slice. Stick a toothpick into each banana "sandwich" and freeze for 30 minutes.
3. Melt the chocolate chips in a double boiler on the stove, or microwave on high for 1 minute, stir well, and then microwave again until the chocolate is melted.
4. Dip the bananas in the chocolate or drizzle it on top. Roll in the coconut flakes and freeze for at least an hour. Remove from the freezer 5 minutes before serving.

BETTER PEANUT BUTTER CUPS

There is something magical about the chocolate and peanut butter combination, but store-bought versions are not the healthiest. This dessert is incredibly easy to make and way better for you. Try not to eat all of these at once!

INGREDIENTS (10 Servings):

1 cup semisweet chocolate chips
1 cup organic peanut butter
1 tablespoon raw honey
½ teaspoon sea salt
1 teaspoon pure vanilla extract

DIRECTIONS:

1. Melt the chocolate chips in a double boiler on the stove, or microwave on high for 1 minute, stir well, and then microwave again until the chocolate is melted.
2. Using a spoon or clean pastry brush, coat 10 silicone candy molds with a thin layer of chocolate.
3. Freeze the molds for 15 minutes, then remove from the freezer and add another thin coat of chocolate. Freeze for another 15 minutes.
4. Mix the peanut butter, honey, salt, and vanilla together in a bowl. Spoon or pipe a big dollop of the mixture into the center of each chocolate cup.
5. Add the remaining melted chocolate on top of the peanut butter mixture (returning the chocolate to the stove or microwave to remelt, if necessary) and freeze for another 15 minutes, then enjoy!

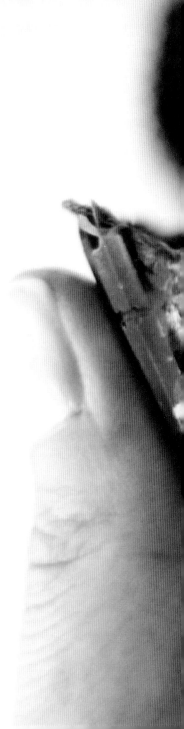

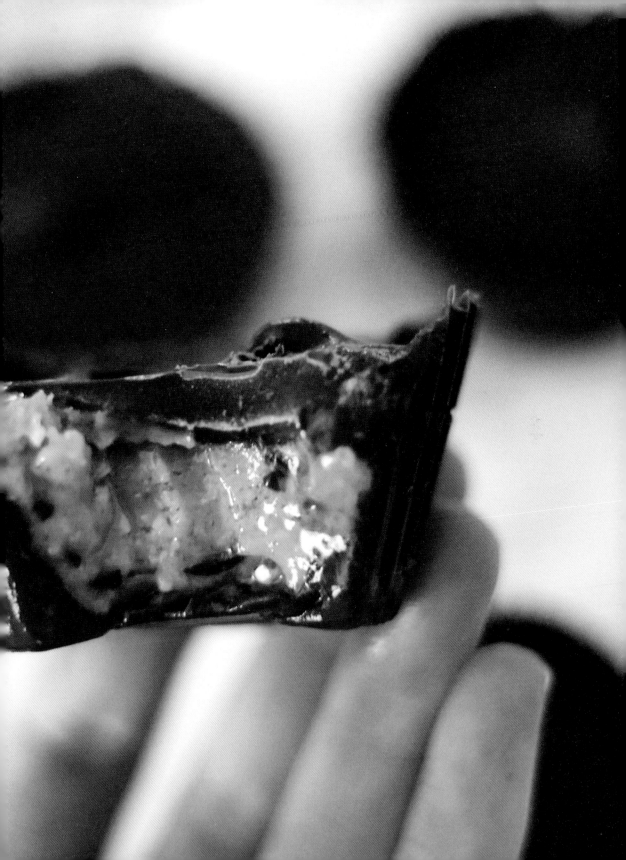

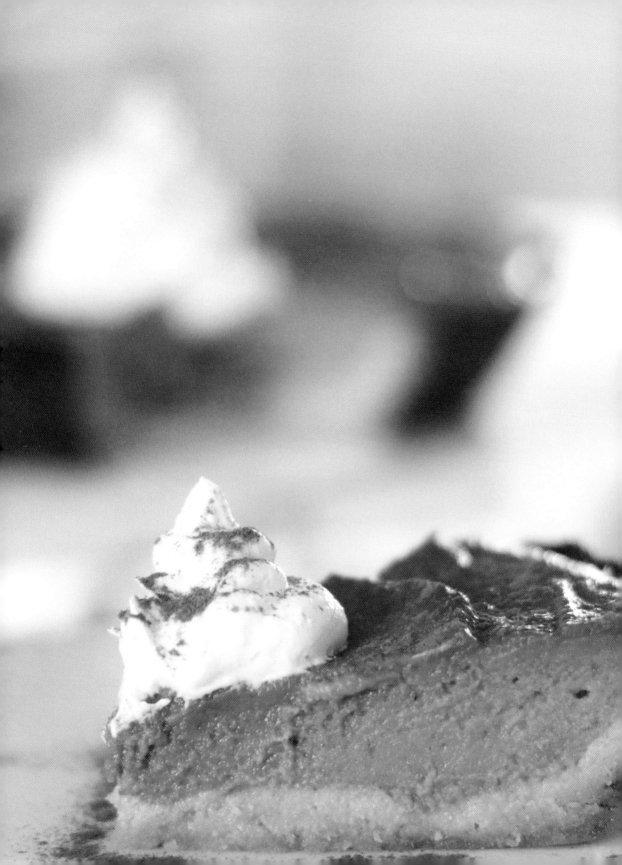

PALEO PUMPKIN PIE

Pumpkin pie is such a classic comfort food during cool weather! This one provides delicious taste without the guilt. It's dairy-free, gluten-free, and nutrient-dense because of the coconut oil, pumpkin, and spices.

INGREDIENTS (8 Servings):

CRUST

2 cups almond meal

1 organic pasture-raised egg

1 tablespoon coconut oil

1 tablespoon raw honey or agave syrup

¼ teaspoon pure vanilla extract

FILLING

1 (15-ounce) can organic pumpkin puree

½ cup full-fat coconut milk

¼ cup raw honey or agave syrup

3 organic pasture-raised eggs

½ teaspoon pure vanilla extract

1 teaspoon pumpkin pie spice

1 teaspoon ground cinnamon

¼ teaspoon ground turmeric

¼ teaspoon freshly ground black pepper

¼ teaspoon maca powder

DIRECTIONS:

CRUST

1. Preheat the oven to 350°F.
2. Combine the crust ingredients in a food processor and pulse until fully mixed. Press the crust evenly into a pie dish and bake for 10 minutes.

FILLING

1. Lightly pulse the filling ingredients together in a blender. This step is important so that you do not whip the eggs. You can also blend the pumpkin, coconut milk, honey, vanilla, and spices by hand, then lightly beat in the eggs one at a time until combined.
2. Pour the filling into the crust and bake for 40 minutes. The center most likely will not be fully set at this point.
3. Refrigerate for 1 hour to set. Bring to room temperature before serving.

"Because of the years of hard-core restricting, I started eating when I was lonely, stressed, etc. Now I have a very healthy relationship with food, exercise, and my body and have been able to make a career out of teaching others about this as an author, business consultant, health coach, yoga teacher, and lifestyle blogger."

RAW VEGAN CHEESECAKE BARS

I'm dessert obsessed, and this is one of my favorite recipes. Colorful and nutritious, these cheesecake slices are always just the thing for any occasion!

INGREDIENTS (30 Servings):

½ cup almond meal

½ packed cup pitted Medjool dates

¾ teaspoon sea salt, divided

½ teaspoon ground turmeric

1 cup cashews, soaked in water overnight and rinsed well

Juice of 1 lemon

¼ cup plus 1 tablespoon pure maple syrup, divided

¼ cup extra-virgin coconut oil, melted

1 teaspoon pure vanilla extract

1 teaspoon maca powder

1–3 tablespoons water, as needed

1 cup blueberries

½ cup strawberries

Toppings: unsweetened coconut flakes, cacao nibs, sliced
    strawberries

DIRECTIONS:

1. In a food processor, combine the almond meal, dates, ¼ teaspoon of the salt, and turmeric. Pulse continuously until a dough forms. Line an ⅛-size sheet pan (9 1/2 x 6 1/2) or other small pan with plastic wrap and press the dough into it evenly, forming a crust.

2. Place the cashews, lemon juice, ¼ cup of the maple syrup, coconut oil, vanilla, remaining ½ teaspoon salt, and maca powder in a food processor and blend until completely smooth, scraping the sides as necessary. Drizzle a little water in slowly, 1 tablespoon at a time, until a creamy consistency is achieved.

3. Pour three-fourths of the mixture onto the crust and freeze for 10 minutes. Add the blueberries to the remaining cheesecake mixture and blend until fully combined. Add this to one half of the cheesecake, leaving the other half with just the original bottom layer.

4. Blend the strawberries with the remaining 1 tablespoon maple syrup. Add dollops of the strawberry mixture with a spoon to the plain side of the cheesecake, then drag a knife blade through the dollops to create a swirl pattern. Top with coconut flakes, cacao nibs, and sliced strawberries. Freeze for at least 2 hours.

5. Allow to thaw for 10 to 15 minutes before serving.

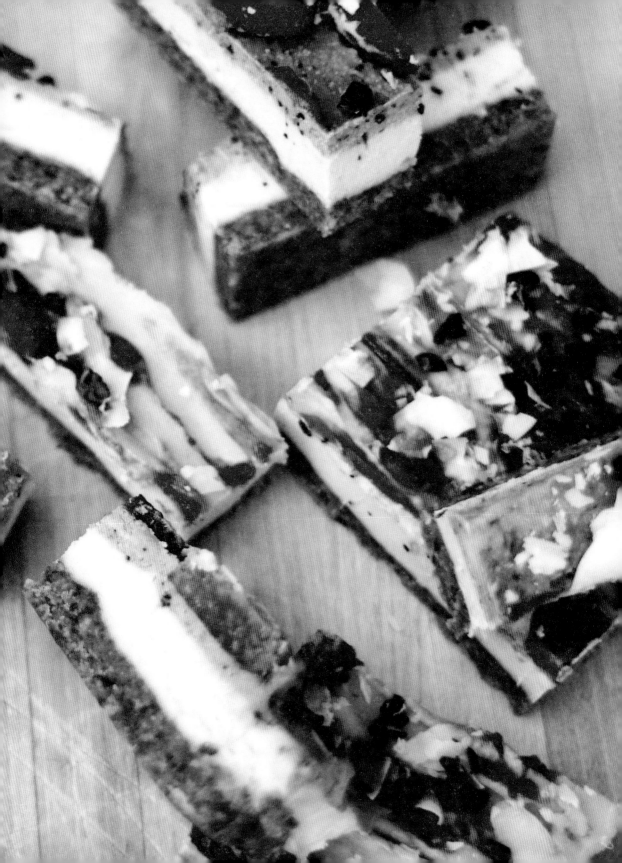

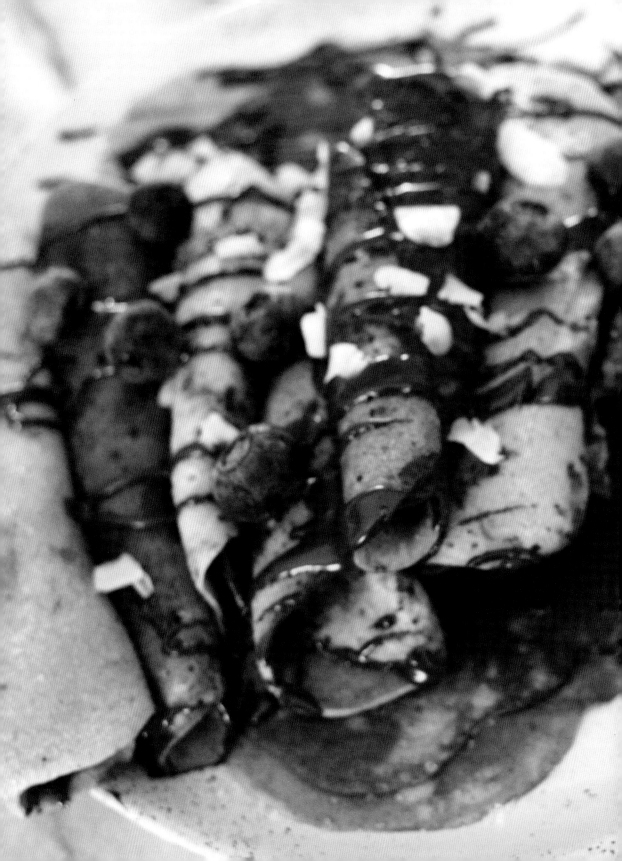

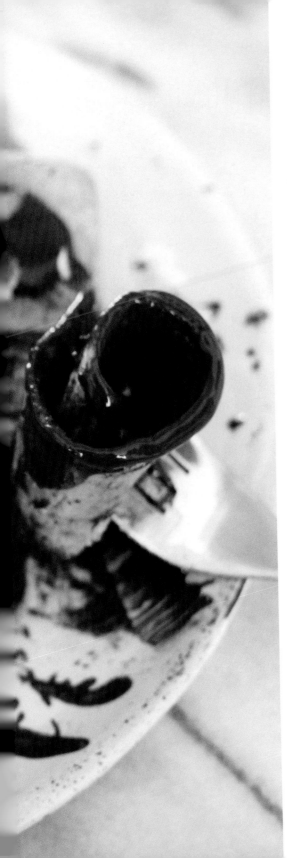

HEALTHIER CHOCOLATE CREPES

These crepes are a family favorite, as they contain healthy ingredients like oats and coconut nectar, instead of the typical white flour and sugar. They won't spike your blood sugar like most breakfast dishes but will satisfy any sweet tooth. Paired with dark chocolate, they're great for a weekend brunch.

INGREDIENTS (1 Serving):

1 cup oat flour
2 large organic pasture-raised eggs
¼ cup water
1 tablespoon coconut nectar
¼ teaspoon pure vanilla extract
1 tablespoon coconut oil
¼ cup semisweet chocolate chips, for sauce
Optional toppings: fresh fruit, nuts

DIRECTIONS:

1. Blend the oat flour, eggs, water, coconut nectar, and vanilla in a blender or food processor until smooth.

2. In a skillet, heat the coconut oil over medium-high heat. Pour about ¼ cup of the batter onto the center of the pan and spread quickly so the crepe is very thin. Cook for 2 minutes, or until the bottom is brown, then flip. Repeat the process until the batter is gone.

3. Melt the chocolate chips in a cup in the microwave or in a small pot over low heat, taking care not to scorch the chocolate.

4. Drizzle the chocolate over the crepes, roll into tubes, and serve immediately. Top with fruit and nuts if desired.

PALEO COOKIES 'N' ALMOND MYLK

Cookies and milk—there's something about this combination that brings you back to childhood and makes you feel warm and grounded. Yet so many cookies out there are high in sugar and additives and contain flours that upset the stomach. These cookies use almond flour, which is easily digestible, and will leave you wanting more. They have become a staple in my kitchen, as I whip them together and eat them with a tall glass of homemade almond mylk any time I'm craving something sweet.

INGREDIENTS (10 Cookies):

COOKIES

2 cups almond flour

½ teaspoon baking soda

½ teaspoon salt

¼ cup coconut oil, melted

2 teaspoons pure vanilla extract

3 tablespoons Grade B maple syrup

¼ cup cacao nibs or dark chocolate chips

Optional: sea salt flakes

ALMOND MYLK

1 cup almonds, soaked in water overnight and rinsed well

2 cups water

1 teaspoon pure vanilla extract (optional)

Pinch of sea salt (optional)

1 Medjool date, pitted (optional)

DIRECTIONS:

COOKIES

1. Preheat the oven to 350°F. Line a baking sheet with parchment paper or a silicone baking mat.
2. In a large mixing bowl, combine the almond flour, baking soda, and salt. Add the melted coconut oil, vanilla, and maple syrup, and mix well.
3. Gently stir in the cacao nibs.
4. Use a spoon to scoop roughly a tablespoon of dough, then place on the baking tray. I like to pat the top down so that they bake into a thinner and rounder cookie, but this is optional. To make these cookies even more decadent, add a pinch of sea salt flakes to the top of each.
5. Bake for 8 to 10 minutes, then remove and let cool.

ALMOND MYLK

1. In a blender, blend the almonds with the water, then strain with a nut milk bag.
2. Optionally, re-blend the milk with the vanilla, a pinch of salt, and a pitted date to sweeten.

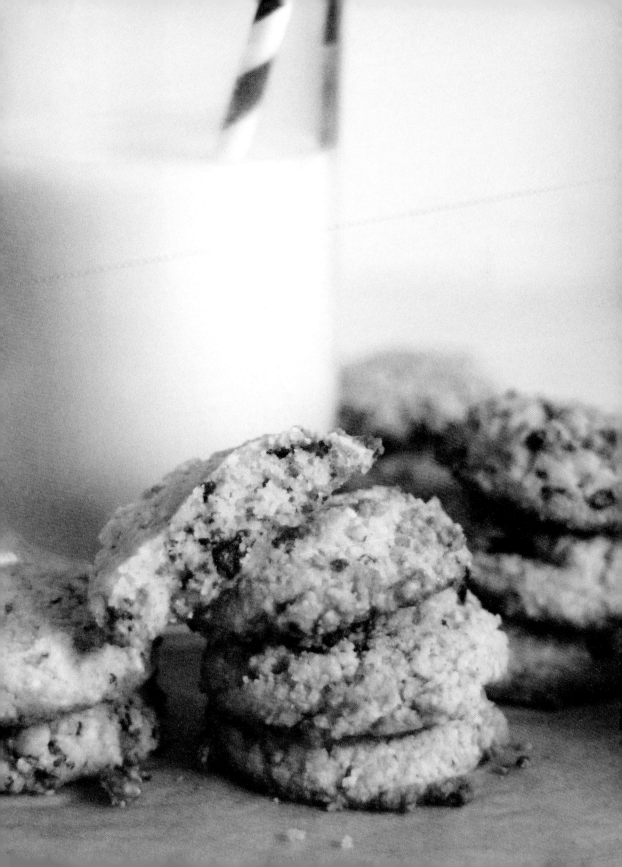

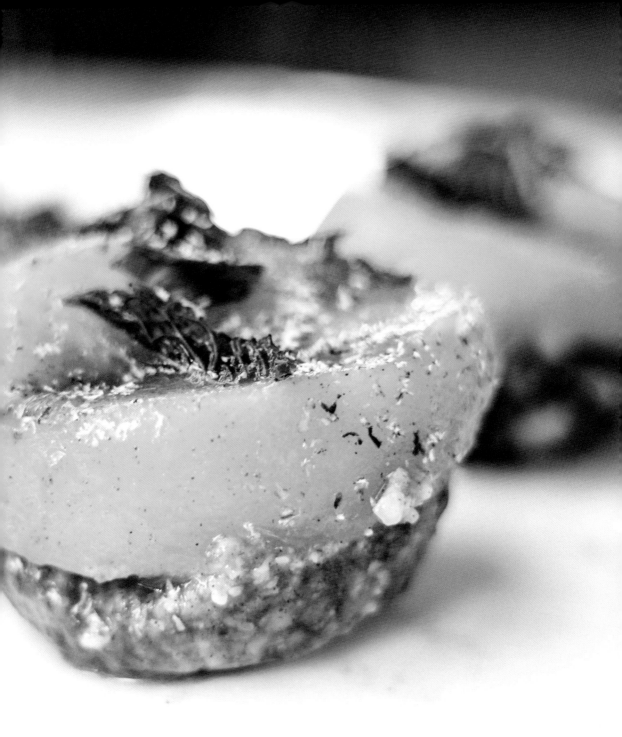

DECONSTRUCTED RAW PEACH COBBLER

This is a deconstructed version of a cobbler, and it's absolutely delicious. It's light and fresh and will have you wanting to eat it all. I like to add mint for an extra pop of color and nutrition, plus it pairs wonderfully with the peaches and lemon. This dessert is fully raw and it's safe to say you won't even miss the original version.

INGREDIENTS (4 Servings):

CRUST

6 Medjool dates, pitted and soaked in water

½ cup almonds

2 teaspoons ground cinnamon

½ teaspoon pure vanilla extract

¼ cup walnuts

COBBLER

2 peaches, pitted

Juice of 1 lemon

1 teaspoon ground cinnamon, plus more for dusting

1 scant tablespoon raw honey or agave syrup

½ teaspoon pure vanilla extract

¼ teaspoon grated nutmeg

Small handful fresh mint, for garnish

DIRECTIONS:

CRUST

1. Blend the crust ingredients in a food processor or high-speed blender until combined but slightly chunky.
2. Press the crust evenly into the bottom of 4 cupcake-size silicone molds and freeze for 2 hours.

COBBLER

1. Cut the peaches into thin slices. Mix the peaches with the lemon juice, cinnamon, honey, vanilla, and nutmeg and set aside for 10 minutes to combine.
2. Top the crust with the cobbler mix, dust with cinnamon, and garnish with mint.

CANDY CORN PARFAIT

Sweet, bright candy corn makes this healthy confection a celebration of autumn, but you can enjoy it any time of year. Orange and pineapple are beautifully complemented by creamy coconut milk.

INGREDIENTS (2 Servings):

3 clementines or 2 navel oranges, peeled and split into
   sections
1 cup diced pineapple
1 (14-ounce) can unsweetened full-fat coconut milk,
   refrigerated overnight or for at least 4 hours
¼ teaspoon pure vanilla extract
1 teaspoon raw honey
Optional toppings: coconut flakes, candy corn

DIRECTIONS:

1. Line the bottom of each of two clear stemless glasses or small mason jars with the orange pieces, and layer the pineapple evenly over the orange layer.

2. To make whipped cream, remove the can of coconut milk from the refrigerator, flip it upside down, and open from the bottom end. Drain the liquid (save for smoothies or other recipes) and scoop the solid coconut milk into a bowl.

3. Add the vanilla and honey and whip with an electric hand mixer or whisk until fluffy whipped cream forms. Scoop a large spoonful on top of each glass, then top with the coconut flakes and candy corn (if using).

Note: The candy corn is not a healthy option, but if you are trying to go for a balanced lifestyle, using a few of them for this parfait is okay. For optimum nutrition, instead add chopped nuts of choice.

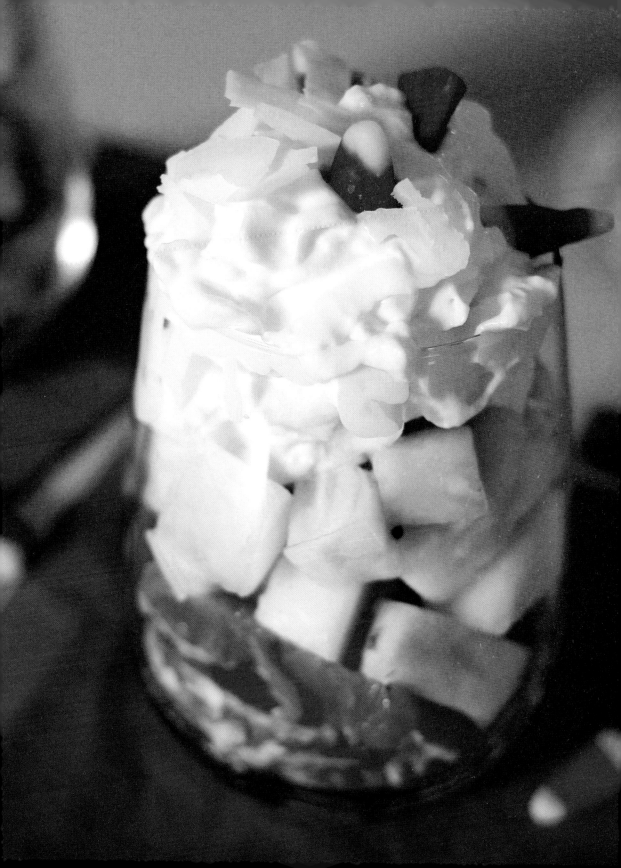

Liquid Recipes

BY JILL DE JONG

Everything you put in your mouth is going to influence how you feel. This chapter is designed to make you feel great! Just pick how you'd like to feel, follow the instructions, and enjoy. These liquid recipes deliver a powerful dose of delicious nutrition, while hydrating your body and satisfying your cravings. So go ahead—drink up!

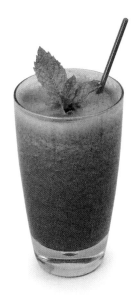

SWEET

Sweet summer fruits combined with icy cool mint make for a deliciously refreshing drink that you can enjoy anytime, especially on hot days.

INGREDIENTS (1 Serving):

1½ cups cubed watermelon
½ orange, peeled
½ cup pineapple chunks
3 ice cubes
1 fresh mint leaf

DIRECTIONS:

1. Combine all the ingredients in a powerful blender and blend until smooth.

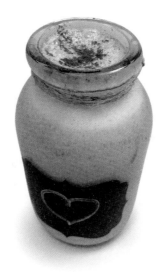

DREAMY

Creamy, dreamy coconut flakes are blended with naturally sweet dates, and then strained for a smooth concoction that's tempered by delicious vanilla and just a hint of sea salt.

INGREDIENTS (1 Serving):

½ cup coconut milk

1½ cups water

2 Medjool dates, pitted

¾ teaspoon pure vanilla extract

¼ teaspoon ground cinnamon

Tiny pinch of sea salt

DIRECTIONS:

1. Combine all the ingredients in a powerful blender and blend until smooth.
2. Serve over ice (don't blend it in).

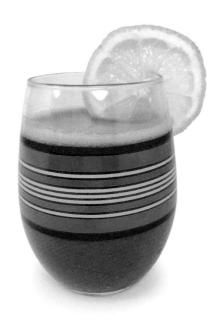

REFRESHED

The classic combination of bright, juicy strawberries and cooling basil gets a citrusy boost from tart lemon and a hint of sweetness from agave syrup or honey.

INGREDIENTS (1 Serving):

½ cup frozen strawberries

1½ cups water

2 teaspoons raw agave or raw honey

½ lemon, peeled

½ cup chopped basil

DIRECTIONS:

1. Combine all the ingredients in a powerful blender and blend until smooth.

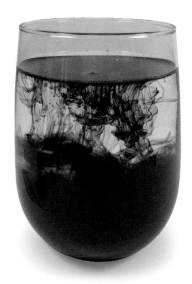

ENERGIZED

Extracted from nettle leaves, ChlorOxygen is a chlorophyll supplement that helps support a healthy liver, builds red blood cells, and can even help with altitude sickness.

INGREDIENTS (1 Serving):

ChlorOxygen liquid
1¼–1½ cups water

DIRECTIONS:

1. Add 15 to 35 drops of ChlorOxygen, per label instructions, to a glass of water and stir. Avoid contact with clothes, as the liquid will permanently stain fabric.

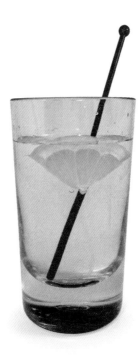

CLEANSED

Apple cider vinegar and lemon juice, two detoxing powerhouses, are mixed together in a simple water blend that hydrates the body while cleansing it internally.

INGREDIENTS (1 Serving):

½ lemon

1¼–1½ cups water

1 teaspoon raw unfiltered apple cider vinegar

DIRECTIONS:

1. Squeeze the lemon juice into the water, add the apple cider vinegar, and stir.

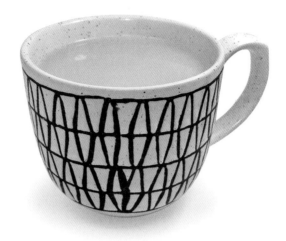

PRODUCTIVE

Yerba mate, a South American tea, is rich in antioxidants, polyphenols, and caffeine. This wondrous herb has many health benefits, including preventing cancer, improving digestion, and strengthening the heart.

INGREDIENTS (1 Serving):

1 yerba mate tea bag

1¼–1½ cups hot water

1–2 teaspoons raw honey

Splash of milk (dairy or plant-based)

DIRECTIONS:

1. Steep the tea bag in the hot water according to package instructions. Add the honey and milk to taste and drink while still warm.

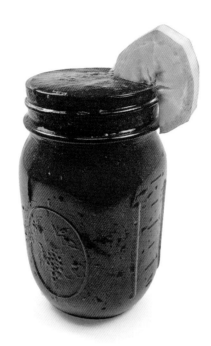

BEAUTIFUL

Fragrant raspberries, sweet banana, nourishing beet, and the tangy sweetness of pineapple make this concoction as delicious as it is beautifying. Beets detoxify the skin while slowing the aging process, and anthocyanins in raspberries are essential for a glowing, youthful complexion.

INGREDIENTS (1 Serving):

1 cup water
½ beet, steamed
1 cup frozen raspberries
1 frozen banana
2 slices pineapple

DIRECTIONS:

1. Combine all the ingredients in a powerful blender and blend until smooth.

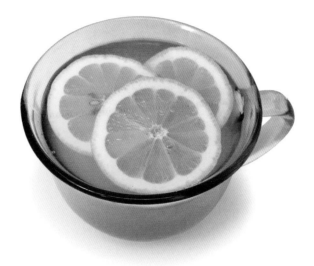

HEALED

Spicy, vibrant turmeric, of the ginger family, is not just for curries. This anti-inflammatory root has long been prized for its healing properties. This drink will help boost immunity, relieve headaches, and prevent muscle soreness after hard workouts.

INGREDIENTS (1 Serving):

1–2 teaspoons raw honey
Juice of ½ lemon
¼ teaspoon ground turmeric
1½ cups hot water

DIRECTIONS:

1. Add the honey, fresh lemon juice, and turmeric powder to the hot water and stir until blended.

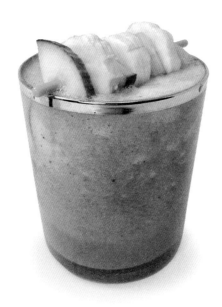

COOL

Be cool as a cucumber with this soothing, tangy tonic made with sweet, delicious pineapple and banana. Cucumbers provide phytonutrients that promote wellness, while bananas provide potassium and pineapples boost immunity, support eye health, and contain antioxidants.

INGREDIENTS (1 Serving):

1 cup sliced cucumber

1 cup chopped pineapple, fresh or frozen

½ banana

¾ cup water

DIRECTIONS:

1. Combine all the ingredients in a powerful blender and blend until smooth. Serve over ice.

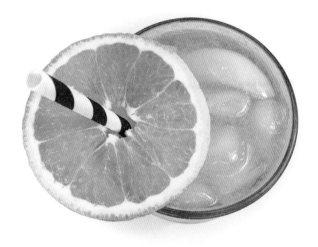

BUBBLY

Orange juice isn't just for the breakfast table! The next time you find yourself craving a sugary soda, reach for this healthier option instead. Orange juice is rich in vitamin C and other nutrients and can help prevent disease and boost the immune system.

INGREDIENTS (1 Serving):

1–2 teaspoons raw agave syrup
Juice of 1 orange
1¼–1½ cups sparkling water

DIRECTIONS:

1. Stir the raw agave and orange juice into the sparkling water.

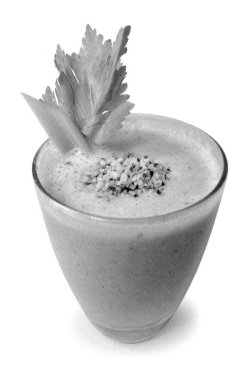

LIGHT

Grab a quick burst of fruity energy and healthy fat and protein with this delicious combination of banana and hemp seeds. Hydrating celery adds essential vitamins and minerals to this tasty tonic. Toss in a pitted date for added sweetness. For a creamier drink, freeze the banana before blending.

INGREDIENTS (1 Serving):

1½ cups water
1 banana
1 celery stalk
3 tablespoons hemp seeds
1 Medjool date, pitted
3–4 ice cubes (optional)

DIRECTIONS:

1. Combine all the ingredients in a powerful blender and blend until smooth.

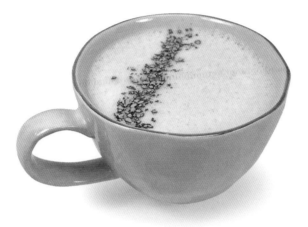

COZY

Matcha, a powdered green tea, is plentiful in antioxidants, chlorophyll, and polyphenols. Mix with milk and honey for a richly comforting drink without the guilt.

INGREDIENTS (1 Serving):

1 cup milk (dairy or plant-based)
1 teaspoon matcha powder
½ cup water
Raw honey, to taste

DIRECTIONS:

1. For the best results, blend the milk and matcha powder in a blender. Combine the milk mixture and water in a small pan and bring to a boil over medium-high heat. Stir in the honey, to taste.
2. If you don't blend the matcha and milk first, then combine just the milk and water in a small pan and bring to a boil over medium-high heat. Whisk in the matcha powder until thoroughly dissolved and then stir in the honey, to taste.

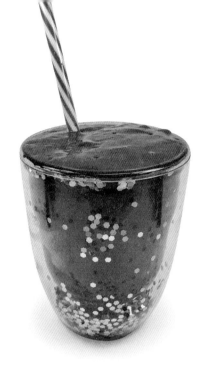

GLORIOUS

Connect to your female power with this nourishing smoothie. The avocado and frozen banana deliver a heavenly creaminess, while maca, an ancient herb that promotes sexual health and improves fertility, adds an extra nutritional punch.

INGREDIENTS (1 Serving):

1 orange, peeled

1 banana, peeled and frozen

1 (3.5 ounce) package unsweetened frozen acai berry puree

1 cup almond milk

1 teaspoon maca powder

¼ avocado

Pinch of ground turmeric (optional)

DIRECTIONS:

1. Place the orange, banana, acai berry puree, almond milk, maca powder, and avocado in a high-speed blender and blend until smooth.
2. Sprinkle with ground turmeric (if using) and serve.

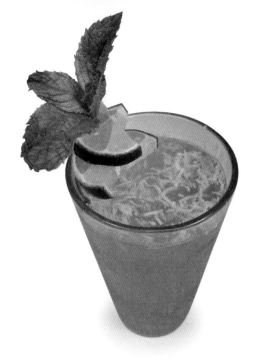

ELEVATED

If you love a cold ginger ale on a hot summer day, but not the sugar and inevitable sugar crash that comes with it, you'll be happy to know it's very easy to make a healthier version at home. Freshly grated ginger makes this lightly sweetened thirst quencher a refreshing beverage that is medicine for the body.

INGREDIENTS (1 Serving):

½ teaspoon finely grated fresh ginger
Juice of ½ lime
1–2 teaspoons agave syrup
1½–2 cups sparkling water

DIRECTIONS:

1. Combine the ginger, lime juice, and agave in a glass, then pour in the sparking water. Give it a good stir with a fork and enjoy.

Afterword

Gone are the days when people starved themselves to look good. Thanks to a better knowledge of nutrition, we can have our cake and eat it too, as long as the cake is made with wholesome ingredients and nourishes the body. This is possible when we replace processed foods that contain added chemicals and refined sugar with better quality unprocessed alternatives, which is exactly what *Models Do Eat* brings us!

I was born in 1987, and when I was growing up as a teenager, it was "cool" to be really thin, with no curves, so we starved ourselves. My story of hitting rock bottom with my health and suffering from a list of health issues, and then transforming it to experience a kind of health I never knew was possible, is in my books. We are witnessing a very exciting time in history, this health revolution, where now it's cooler to be healthy, not stick thin, and what's trending is nourishing green juices, smoothies, and natural desserts.

This book is for you if you are looking for delicious comfort food that won't harm your health. Thanks to my own disordered eating, I did tremendous damage to my health and body as a teen. But since pledging myself to this natural lifestyle, my health and figure have bounced back. These recipes will change your life and transform your health, as many others around the world have already discovered.

Models Do Eat is for you if you are looking for the freedom to fully embrace and enjoy the rest of your life, especially if you suffer from any eating disorders, including binge eating, junk food addiction, overeating, bulimia, anorexia, emotional eating, and generally disordered eating.

This book will help you regain your self-worth so that you will know your value. It will help you embrace your beauty, both inside and out. It will help you break through any self-limiting beliefs and thoughts you may have about yourself.

Jill de Jong is truly one of the healthiest and

most vibrant human beings I have ever met. In my travels to seventeen countries and all fifty U.S. states, I have met tens of thousands of people. Jill stands out to me as a woman who embodies wholesome health in mind, body, and spirit. When we walk down the street together, everyone looks at her; her height and outer beauty are obvious to all who can see. But then when people get to know her, they quickly learn she is a beautiful soul with a pure heart. She did such a great job in putting this book together to assist others in transforming their health and lives!

Enjoy the lifesaving recipes and life-changing tips in this book and help us spread the word that "models do eat." The only way to have a happy life is to be healthy, and when we are healthy on the inside, it always shows on the outside. This book will teach you how to enjoy living in your dream body!

— Liana Werner-Gray,
best-selling author of *The Earth Diet*
and *10-Minute Recipes*

Acknowledgments

"When one door closes, another door opens."

I'd like to start with a big thank you to the publishing houses that rejected this project the first time it was reviewed. It changed my life in the best possible way: it propelled me to get certified as a health coach and personal trainer, and this book turned into a wonderful book collaboration instead.

Eleonora, you did a great job selecting the best agents for this project.

Maura and the Don Congdon Associates, thank you for believing in me and taking this project to the publishing houses not once but twice!

Abigail, I couldn't have done this without you. All the countless hours we worked on this were so worth it.

Liana, you've always believed that this book was going to be published. Your encouragement and excitement have helped me push through.

Taylor, Nikki, CJ, Summer, Liana, Lauren, Sarah, Adela, and Colleen, I'm so grateful that you shared your stories, passion, and recipes in this book. I'm proud of us!

BenBella, thanks for giving me the opportunity to share this heartfelt project with the world. It's a dream come true.

The BenBella team, especially Trish, Leah, and Jessika, you've all been so easy to work with. Thanks for your diligence, patience, and hard work!

Much gratitude to my parents, Tryntsje and Hilbrand, for raising me with wholesome foods and strong values.

Eric, I love your excitement for every meal we make and eat together. You are so sweet.

And last but not least, I'd like to thank my closest friends for their love and support.

Life is better shared. To many more yummy meals and meaningful conversations.

Big hugs,

— Jill

Photo Credits

Photos on pages 13 and 41 by Greg Hinsdale

Collage photography on page 42: Eduardo Von Garcia—www.eduardovongarcia.com (center), Riker Brothers (bottom right) and Jill de Jong (remainder)

Photo on page 43 by Greg Hinsdale

Photo on page 47 courtesy of Jill de Jong

Protein Power recipe photography by Jill de Jong

Collage photography on page 60: Mario Machado Photography (top right, center, bottom right), Lucca Lowenthal (bottom left), Judy Walker (top left), and Taylor Walker Sinning (remainder)

Photo on page 61 courtesy of Taylor Walker Sinning

Photo on page 67 by Mario Machado Photography

Less Sugar, More Spice recipe photography by Taylor Walker Sinning

Collage photography on page 78: Justin Macala (center), © 2017 Cody Rasmussen | www.codyras.com (bottom right), and Courtney James (remainder)

Photos on pages 79 and 89 courtesy of Courtney James

Paleo Party recipe photography by Courtney James

Collage photography on page 98: Tatiana Katkova (bottom right), Michelle Layne Lawson (top center, bottom center), Marysol Yoo (top left), Kate Moore Photography (center), and Lauren Williams (remainder)

Photo on page 99 by Caley Dimmock

Simply Delicious recipe photography by Michelle Layne Lawson

Photo on page 110 by Caley Dimmock

Collage photography on page 116: Ben Horton Photography (top left, top right, bottom left), Jenna Ohnemus Peffley (center), Rochelle Brodin Photo | @rochellebrodinphoto | Facebook @RochelleBrodinStudio (bottom right), and Colleen Baxter (remainder)

Photo on page 117 © Gina Falcone

Happy Belly recipe photography by Colleen Baxter

Photo on page 124 by Ben Horton Photography

Collage photography on page 134: Benedikt Renc for *Elle Magazine* (center), Photographer: Lucie Robinson | Magazine: *Zen Magazine* (top right), and Adela Capova (remainder)

Photos on pages 135 and 139 by Bradley Ennis

Fitness Fuel recipe photography by Adela Capova

Collage photography on page 154: ©Roxxelreland (top left, center left, bottom center) and Liana Werner-Grey (remainder)

Photos on page 155 and 164 by Derrick Salters/ WENN

Unhealthy Foods Made Healthy recipe photography on pages 157, 158, 162, and 170 ©Roxxelreland. Photography on pages 161, 162, 169 and 173 by Liana Werner-Grey

Collage photography on page 174 and Mostly Plants recipe photography by Summer Rayne Oakes

Photos on pages 175 and 180 by Jonathan Dennish

Collage photography on page 188: SweetEscape | Donny Wu (bottom right), Tamara Muth King (center), Ray Kachatorian (top right), and Nikki Sharp (remainder)

Photos on pages 189 and 195 by Tamara Muth King

Sweets and Treats recipe photography by Nikki Sharp

Liquid Recipes photography by Jill de Jong

Back cover photography: (clockwise)

Summer Rayne Oakes headshot by Jonathan Dennish

Courtney James headshot courtesy of Courtney James

Sarah DeAnna headshot by Phira Luon

Colleen Baxter headshot by Jenna Ohnemus Peffle

Lauren Williams headshot by Caley Dimmock

Nikki Sharp headshot by Tamara Muth King

Taylor Walker Sinning headshot courtesy of Taylor Walker Sinning

Liana Werner-Grey headshot by Derrick Salters/ WENN

Adela Capova headshot by Bradley Ennis

Index

About the Author

Jill de Jong was born in Holland, and her successful modeling career brought her to the United States. She was based in New York for many years, explored Miami for a few years, and then fell in love with Los Angeles, where she currently resides; it's a great place to pursue her passion for health and wellness. After making the career shift from full-time modeling to health coach, personal trainer, and chef, she's never looked back.

When Jill is not working, you can find her in the kitchen cooking or outside in Malibu running, biking, surfing, or stretching in a yoga class. She recharges by spending time with her boyfriend and friends. Meaningful conversations and delicious food make her heart sing. To stay motivated to exercise, she signs up for triathlons and Spartan races.